ACCO

"Rani St. Pucchi's designs are absolutely beautiful!—Thank you!"

—*Alison Krauss,* Singer-Songwriter

"I can't tell you how privileged I feel to wear one of your gowns. You are so talented."

—*Candice Crawford,*
Mrs. Tony Romo, Quarterback, Dallas Cowboys

"I've gone to countless awards and worn countless dresses, but nothing compares to your designs. I got the inspiration for my entire event from my St. Pucchi dress."

—*Sanya Richards-Ross,* Olympic Gold Medalist

"The most incredible designer in the world!"

—*Tara Reid,* Actress

"Rani St. Pucchi is an experienced and gifted designer, an innovator, a pioneer. She is exactly what we need: we need wisdom, we need people who, like Rani, open up their experience and let people learn by sharing it. We hear that women need inspiration, we hear that women need power that they can see in other women, to have confidence in themselves. Rani has a deep understanding of how powerful it is to be elegant and classic and proves that dressing your best lends power and shows security in self."

—*Edward* Tyll,
RADIO PERSONALITY AND HOST OF THE SYNDICATED
RADIO SHOW *THE ED TYLL SHOW.*

"Rani wonderfully illustrates how to dress for your body type. The concepts shared in *Your Body, Your Style* will help women create a positive and powerful self-confidence that will immediately alter the dynamics of their relationships with themselves and with others."

—*Walt Shepard,* FOUNDER AND PUBLISHER, *INSIDE WEDDINGS*

"Written by a true expert, *Your Body, Your Style* goes beyond the trends to help women define their own individual style. Fashion is everywhere we look. It's all around us each and every day. Personal style is intimate. It gives you the inspiration to be free of convention—to express your view of the world and the way in which the world should see you. *Your Body, Your Style* is a comfortable fit for every woman."

—*Jim Duhe,* VP/ASSOCIATE PUBLISHER,
BRIDAL GUIDE MAGAZINE

"*Your Body, Your Style* is much more than a fabulous fashion guide, it is an inspiration! Rani St. Pucchi writes with passion of loving yourself, embracing and accepting your body, which takes courage. Courage is standing up for yourself. It never goes out of style. Empower yourself; read this book!"

—*Val Orr*, FILMMAKER AND AUTHOR *BARNONE*

"*Your Body, Your Style* is a multidimensional book for the fashion-conscious gal, interested in more than a designer label. This is the go-to blueprint for women who know the secret to making an impression comes from the inside out. Rani St. Pucchi's background in design and working with countless fashionistas gives her a unique perspective we can all learn from."

—*Tamra Nashman*, WWW.EXTRA-ORDINARYIMAGE.COM

"*Your Body, Your Style* is simple, yet profound! It's a book of empowerment for women of every age and lifestyle. As Rani points out, empowerment begins with the way we dress our body, and how we develop our unique personal style. A perfect guide for every woman!"

—*RoseLynn Micari-Fiumara*,
OWNER, BRIDAL REFLECTIONS

"This is more than just a book about dressing to flatter our bodies. For me, my body and my style are the secret to my success, balance in life and happiness in my marriage and business. Being able to slip on not just one but more than ten of Rani's delicately elegant dresses took my sleek and sexy style to another level. Style to me is not about being thin or fat, but about dressing and feeling the prettiest you can in the body you have, a healthy attitude and plenty of gratitude. Rani St. Pucchi's *Your Body, Your Style* gives every woman the tools she needs to unlock her femininity."

—Angelle Grace Wacker, SENIOR VICE PRESIDENT, NAI CAPITAL, INC.

"Rani is an amazing designer who truly is in love with fashion. She creates designs that are a second skin and become a calling card for all the lucky women in her world. Her designs speak these powerful words . . . super chic, flirtatious, imaginative. Collections that have a beautiful presence, that speak for your body and give women a glow of confidence, an elegant vision, and a radiant sense of being happy. How we dress and present ourselves is the picture we paint for all to see. Rani's personal spirit, courage & uniqueness is why she has chosen to share with us such intelligent words and give guidance and strength to those who need encouragement. Stylish women are powerful. They are as powerful as a bird in flight when going after their dreams.

Looking and feeling fabulous empowers women to be fabulous! Rani is one of those powerful fabulous women."

—Barbara Tilzer-Frankel, CREATIVE DIRECTOR

"*Your Body, Your Style* is a wonderful book for those who have some knowledge of fashion as well as those who are just beginning to find their way into the fashion world. If you have any questions about finding your way to class, style and a timeless way of designing your look, this book is your answer. Lovely, simple way of learning the tricks of how to dress that flatters every body type. Rani is a first-class designer. I enjoyed this book from beginning to end. Just loved it! You will, too."

—Chanda Montroy, DE LUZ, TEMECULA, CA.

"From dressing for your body type to cleaning out our closets and losing unflattering items, Rani St. Pucchi offers tips for any woman to own her essence and make an impression based on personalized style. I highly recommend *Your Body, Your Style* as a tool to increase self-awareness and enhance self-esteem by owning all that you are from the inside out."

—Lisa Manyon, THE BUSINESS MARKETING ARCHITECT,
WWW.WRITEONCREATIVE.COM

"It's no secret that Rani is one of the most talented fashion designers out there. *Your Body, Your Style* is not just a fashion bible, but it's also a book about accepting your authentic self and working it from there. Thank you, Rani, for synthesizing the world of beauty and practicality to a whole new level for everyone who wants to look AND feel great. You'll be able to refer to this beautiful coffee table gem for many years to come. I look forward to more from Rani!"

—Simran Rajkitkul,
FOUNDER, STORYTIME PRESCHOOL, THAILAND

Your Body, Your Style
by Rani St. Pucchi

© Copyright 2016 Rani St. Pucchi

ISBN 978-0-9976977-1-1

Published by

◤ köehlerbooks™

210 60th Street
Virginia Beach, VA 23451
800-435-4811
www.koehlerbooks.com

Visit us on the web!
www.yourbodyyourstylebook.com
www.ranistpucchi.com

Your BODY Your STYLE

*Simple Tips on
Dressing to Flatter
Your Body Type*

Rani ST. PUCCHI

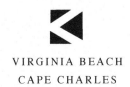

VIRGINIA BEACH
CAPE CHARLES

CONTENTS

CONTENTS

UNLEASH YOUR FEMININITY

It's Time!

Rani St. Pucchi, a trendsetting designer whose expertise has been recognized in such media outlets as *Entertainment Tonight, Harper's Bazaar, WWD, Town and Country, Bride's, Cosmopolitan Bride, Martha Stewart Weddings, and The Knot,* can help define the style that flatters you most—no matter what age or stage of life you are at, or what your body type is.

In this book, Rani shares with you her knowledge of the woman's form and guides you to find simple solutions to your most pressing body concerns. The focus is on you—and how you can make yourself more confident and appealing to others in almost every situation, simply by making a few changes and different choices in planning your wardrobe.

Once you embrace your unique attributes and dissolve your bad relationship to your body, you'll be amazed to find how attractive and irresistible you are to others!

Women from all over the world have clamored to have a private consultation with Rani so they may benefit from her expertise, and with her clear direction and gentle guidance regain their self-confidence and shine. Now you, too, can benefit from her fashion advice.

THIS SIMPLE AND FRIENDLY GUIDE REVEALS:

- What clothes and silhouettes are best for your specific body type
- Simple techniques to determine what colors flatter you most
- Solutions to common lingerie issues and the importance of fit
- The one dress that is a chameleon and how to transform it into different looks
- How to travel stress-free by planning your wardrobe well
- The four-step approach to sort-and-purge, organize, and take control of your wardrobe
- The secrets to shopping smart
- How to define your personal style and embrace your own unique personality
- The 411 on perfumes and why the scent you wear matters
- How to plan a wardrobe for all seasons
- 101 styling secrets, professional tricks, and fashion tips

Rani St. Pucchi is a designer, an author, and a relationship expert. She is a regular contributor to The Huffington Post.

Learn more at www.ranistpucchi.com

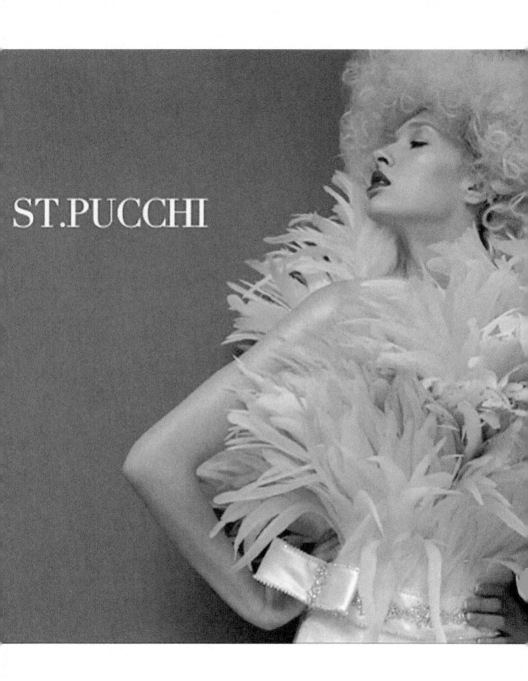

ST.PUCCHI

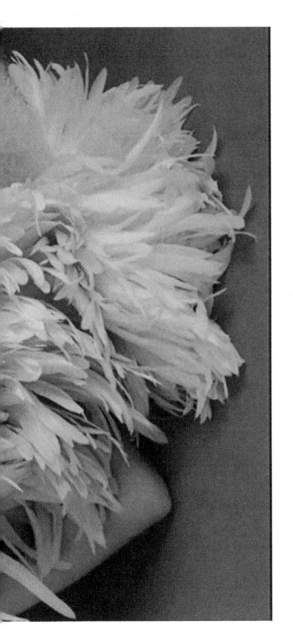

I lovingly dedicate this book to all the women I have had the privilege to meet: those who have been my clients and my friends; those who have been my students and my teachers; those who have shown loving support for my work and who continue to be a source of inspiration to me. My heart has grown so much in knowing each and every one of you.

DEAR BODY

DEAR BODY

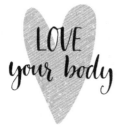

How may I express my love for you?
By promising to be kind to you
By feeding you right and taking care of you lovingly
By dressing you with pride and recognizing your perfection
No matter what anyone else says it doesn't matter
I promise that I will not compare you to any other
You are my strength, my friend, my better half
I vow to see your beauty, your confidence, and your unique personality
I recognize that all body types are beautiful and mine is uniquely mine
My Creator has blessed me with you and I respect and love you.
My standards of beauty and perfection are not determined by any
Because I respect you I give others permission to respect me in kind
I vow to stand up for you and I pledge loyalty until the end of time.

Rani St. Pucchi

INTRODUCTION

I f there is a seminal moment in my relationship to fashion and designing, the occasion that springs to mind is a summer in Bangkok, Thailand. I must have been about four or five years old. My cousin and I were running feverishly from the ground floor of our townhome to my mother's bedroom on the fourth floor to get dressed for the movies, and we were very late.

I looked at the choices I had and was quite disappointed. Even though there were so many options, I kept trying and tossing the frocks one by one on the floor. The cupboard now bare, I hit a wall: I'd run out of clothes. I remember so well the frustration and, at the same time, the aha moment. I decided henceforth I would choose my own fabrics and design my own clothes. After all, who knew better than I what looked good on me?

I thank my parents for drawing me into the magical world of luxury fabrics and laces. As the largest purveyor of fine laces in Thailand, their ateliers and showrooms became my playground where I would spend all my spare time. I had the opportunity to be around fine fabrics and get to touch and feel and know them well. I actively participated with my tailors in transforming these fabrics into unique designs for myself.

Fast-forward to 1984. I was still living in Bangkok, Thailand,

and running my small tailoring shop in a prominent hotel, specializing in ready-to-wear and evening gowns along with men's tailored suits. A rare opportunity came my way when a client asked if I would be willing to bring my collection to showcase at her charity event in San Antonio, Texas.

I was an avid fan of the TV sitcom *Dallas* and always fantasized about living the life of such opulence and outrage as the characters depicted in the series! Traveling to the United States was a dream come true.

With great enthusiasm I prepared a collection of 54 pieces, comprising jackets, skirts, blouses and dresses, and some evening sheaths. As an afterthought, I decided it would be nice to have a finale piece, and so I designed my very first bridal gown for this purpose.

It was a blush-colored wedding gown made of pure Thai silk, entirely hand embroidered and hand beaded. Little did I know that the one wedding gown would receive so much attention as to catapult my whole life!

Next thing I knew I had already committed to showing a bridal collection in Dallas at the Dallas Apparel Mart, which was the go-to fashion platform where buyers from all over the world congregated. I registered my company on a wing and a prayer, and **St. Pucchi** was born.

When I launched my first bridal couture collection at the Dallas Apparel Mart in April of 1985 I was unsure if what I had so lovingly put together was of any value to the US bridal market. I was also clueless to the fact that white was the only color worn and accepted by the American bride at the time.

They say ignorance is bliss! By the time I learned, it was too late. My collection had already shipped from Bangkok to Dallas and there was not a single white dress among the sixteen styles I had designed. The colors ranged from ecru to blush to butterscotch and even pale blue.

I comforted myself into believing that perhaps the US bridal industry as it was could use a fresh perspective and, hopefully, my collection would, at the very least, bring some excitement.

It was pure pleasure to be totally immersed in an unfolding story, on a journey that is never forgotten. My first collection produced in me an intensely emotional and cathartic experience.

After all, I had invested all my resources and used up my credit cards to the max. There was so much riding on my success that I could not fathom what the future would look like if . . .

The Dallas Apparel News ran a front-page story about my premier bridal collection and how it was a harkening of things to come. I was applauded for being a pioneer not only for using pure silks in bridal, which was unheard of at the time, but also for being so bold and daring as to introduce color to bridal wear.

The US bridal industry as we had known it would change forever.

Today, 30-plus years later, with more than 10,000 designs under my belt, I find myself very fortunate and humbled to write this book. The amazing women I've had the pleasure to work with during trunk shows, fashion shows, and on my travels across the globe have taught me much.

I have witnessed again and again how looking good can change a woman's life. I have worked with numerous women, young and old, women getting married, mothers with teenage daughters, women going through midlife crisis and those going through menopause. The story they tell themselves is the same. Most are not happy with their bodies and wish they could change something or the other so they could feel confident in themselves.

A woman's form is the most beautiful, most complex and the most intriguing. Yet we don't appreciate it enough. We tend to hide parts that we feel are not attractive, and we berate ourselves for being too much of this, and not enough of that. Rather than being in awe and working with the form we are blessed with, we spend more time and resources than most of us can afford on diets and procedures that are rarely long lasting.

We're on this constant merry-go-round and obsess about our bodies during every waking moment. Not only that, but the way we talk to ourselves: We would not allow anyone to say those words to our best friends or even our worst enemies!

This book does not pretend to be your road to perfection. The purpose of writing it is to guide you through simple techniques and suggestions on how to look at your body and see what you can make better.

You are asked to assess and appraise your body type so that you can learn about the most flattering silhouettes to dress in.

You will learn how to dress your body in a way that will enhance your best assets and camouflage areas that you feel uncomfortable about or find lacking in any way.

You will realize why it is so important to invest in the right lingerie. You will learn the importance of fit and simple solutions to your common bra issues.

You are invited to learn a simple process to determine what colors flatter you most and which ones to part with. Color is one of the key elements that can make a woman look more interesting, more self-confident, more self-assured, and in control.

You will learn about the one color that is a must-have in every woman's wardrobe, and the one piece of clothing that is a chameleon and that can be transformed into any number of looks.

You are taken on a journey to see how your style and taste evolve as you transition through your 20s, 30s, 40s, 50s, 60s, and beyond. And you learn that sexy is never out of fashion, nor is it outdated. That in fact the older you get the more confident you become. And you realize that ultimately confidence is really what makes a woman sexy.

You become savvy on how and what to pack for your travels, whether you're going on a month-long vacation, a weekend romantic getaway to an exotic tropical island, or a short business trip.

You learn the simple four-step process to sort-and-purge and organize your wardrobe so that no time is wasted in choosing what to wear each day, allowing you time to become more productive in life.

You will learn to plan your shopping sprees wisely and know how to differentiate your wants from your needs.

You will dive into the world of perfumes and learn the intricacies of choosing the perfect scent that resonates with your personality.

You will be able to define your personal style, and become clear on how you wish to be seen in the world. This knowledge will help you embrace your own unique personality and shine.

You will learn to assess and enhance a wardrobe that is suitable for all seasons: fall/winter as well as spring/summer. The checklist of essentials prepares you so you are ready to welcome each season with confidence.

In this book I share 101 tips and tricks on fashion fixes that help you gain self-confidence, tips on how to accentuate your strongest features and dress sexy. You will receive smart shopping hints and simple style advice for your body type and more.

In these pages I share with you the knowledge that I have garnered and reveal those secrets you will now learn so you too can look like a million bucks, regardless of the body you have, or the resources to access trends that are so fleeting they make our heads spin!

Thank you for the opportunity to share my knowledge. I hope it serves you.

Rani St. Pucchi

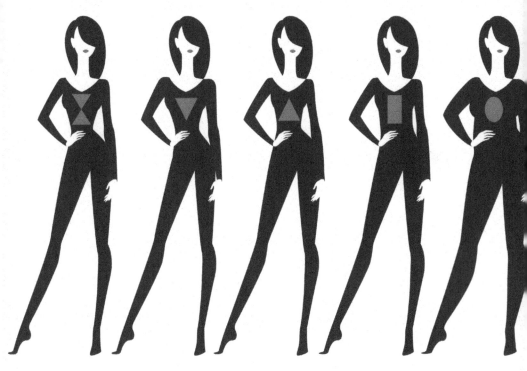

hourglass   inverted triangle   triangle   rectangle   apple

CHAPTER ONE

B ody confidence does not come from trying to achieve the perfect body. It comes from embracing the one you've already got.

What is perfection? What is a perfect body?

Do you hear that voice in your head, the one that is constantly telling you that you can't wear those jeans because your hips look gargantuan in them? That you look ridiculous in that off-the-shoulder number that you swore was the sexiest thing in your wardrobe? Confront it and say: *Do you mean that I'm curvy like Salma Hayek? Petite like Eva Longoria? Tall like Taylor Swift? I'll take that!*

Imperfection is beautiful.

Let the angst go. Rest assured that most of us do not have perfect bodies like those we see in films and magazines. Those are actually Photoshopped—really! And even so-called "perfect" celebrities require some specialized attention to what they wear and how.

The general rule in dressing your best and most flattering is to try and disguise your so-called "defects" and enhance the best attributes of your silhouette.

It would be fabulous to have a perfect body, but the fact is most of us do not. What each one of us does have are different, unique characteristics. The feminine figure cannot be classified easily, but it is possible to generalize certain types of basic silhouettes.

In this chapter you will learn to identify your body shape. Knowing your body type is the first key to knowing how to dress to look your best.

The five basic body types are: Hourglass, Apple, Pear, Ruler, and Inverted Triangle.

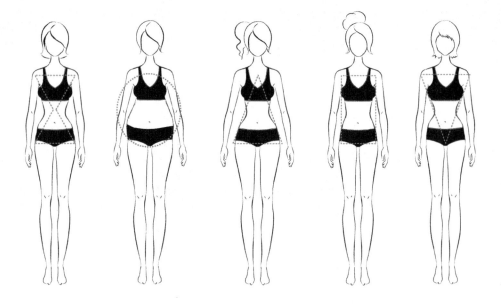

All women lean toward one of these basic shapes, but only a few of us will be exactly one of these. For instance, if your bust or your waist size changes you may get different results.

If you know the measurements of your bust, waist and hips you can also use an online calculator by going to www.calculator.net/body-type-calculator, which will give you a general idea of the body type you fall under.

HOURGLASS

Your hips and bust are usually equal, with a well-defined narrow waist. Fat is generally stored evenly throughout. Your curves are flattering in the right places, although you can still have fleshy upper arms and wide-looking shoulders.

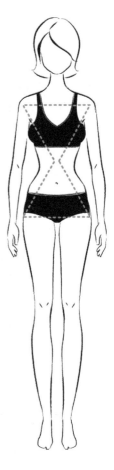

Hourglass

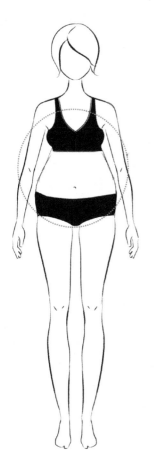

Apple

APPLE

Your bust is a few inches larger than your hips. Your weight is concentrated around your mid-section and chest, sometimes giving the illusion of a bigger bust and a protruding stomach. Your waistline has little definition, and though you are top heavy, your legs tend to be slimmer. Wide shoulders and slim limbs, especially the arms, are the usual characteristics of this body type.

PEAR/TRIANGLE

Described as the most "curvaceous" body of all types. You are the opposite of the apple body type, as you are bottom heavy with hips that are wider than your shoulders. Fat tends to accumulate on your thighs and sometimes the buttocks. Therefore your lower body—hips, thighs, and sometimes your behind—are more noticeable. Your shoulders are narrower, sloping, and not as broad. You tend to have an elongated waist and your legs tend to be shorter and are noticeably wider, muscular, and fuller compared to the rest of your body.

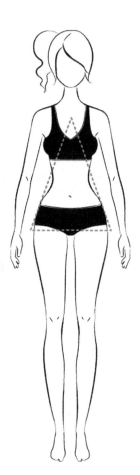

Pear

RULER

Also described as straight/rectangular. The ruler has a "boyish" profile and may have a thin body that tends to lack curves. Your hips tend to have a similar width to your shoulders. Your waist measures about the same as your bust and hips. You cannot notice any significant curves around the waist area and there is no waist definition. Your bust tends to be small or average. You will look fairly straight up with flat shoulders.

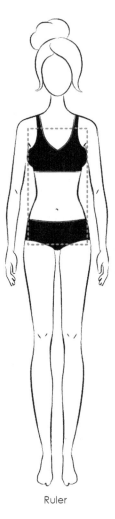

Ruler

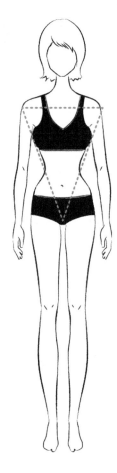

Inverted Triangle

INVERTED TRIANGLE

This is the opposite of the Pear shape. You are top heavy: broader on the top and narrower on the bottom. You usually wear a larger size on top. Your shoulders are wider and broader, your hips narrower. Your bust tends to be proportionately large. Your waist is a few inches smaller than your hips, and your legs are usually slimmer.

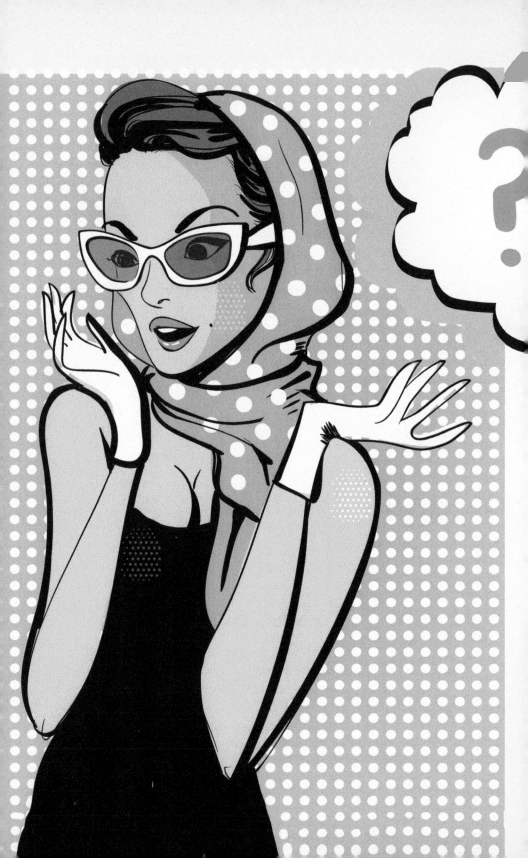

CHAPTER TWO

When choosing your clothes, remember that clothes are meant to flatter your body, not your body to flatter your clothes. Work with your body instead of critiquing and judging it.

Now that you've assessed your body type, let's delve into what would look most flattering and what you would be smart to avoid.

HOURGLASS

The hourglass is seen by many as the ideal body type, although it may present some challenges, particularly if you have a significant bust or if you tend to gain some weight around the abdomen area.

You will want to accentuate your very feminine body, so clothes that are fitted at the right places are key. Another objective maybe to wear clothes that elongate your legs. Focus on your waist when choosing your wardrobe. Dress to flatter your beautiful curves by wearing clothes and accessories that emphasize the thinnest part of your waist. You have admirable curves, so embrace them and show them off.

DO:

- Draw attention to your waistline by wearing belts that cinch the waist.
- V-neck dresses and tops with deep necklines are typically quite flattering.
- Look for dresses that fit your bust and elongate your waist.
- Wear a good supportive bra that will thrust your bust forward.
- If you have some weight around your abdomen then wear shirts and dresses in supportive fabrics.
- T-shirts and tank tops that fit your waist or that have a V-neck and some accents on the shoulders look best.
- Tops that flare from under the bust can be very flattering with pants.
- Coats and jackets that feature V-necklines and are tapered at the waist look best.
- Single-breasted jackets that are tailored look great when left open to create a nice vertical line, elongating your torso.

- Wear darker colors on top if your intention is to make your bust appear smaller.
- Little fitted jackets that tuck in your bust will look great on you.
- Pencil skirts that are tapered help accentuate your wonderful curves.
- Skirts look best when they end at the knee.
- Flat-front boot cut trousers with some stretch for a snug fit are flattering.

DON'T:

- Avoid "boxy" clothes and those that are shapeless or drape-y since they tend to add bulk and make you look heavy.
- Don't go braless when wearing V-neck dresses or tops.
- Avoid shirts that have buttons all the way to the top.
- Avoid too many frills and ruffles, as they will add extra bulk to places where you don't need it.
- Avoid over-complicated styles and excess fabric, as they tend to add bulk.

APPLE

This is perhaps the most challenging body shape to dress, as many women with this shape are well aware of. Because they have no defined waist and weight tends to form on the stomach, many women with this body type tend to cover it all up with loose and unshapely garments. In fact what they ought to focus on is creating the most flattering silhouette possible by creating the illusion of a waist and highlighting their cleavage, as well as wearing clothes with vertical lines to achieve a long and lean look.

DO:

- Make wearing a good-fitting bra a top priority, since much attention is drawn to the top part of your body.

- Direct attention away from your waist by wearing clothes that accentuate your bust and hips instead.

- Wear dresses with waistlines hitting just below the bust or at your thinnest part.

- Wear tops that highlight your body at the slimmest point, which is just underneath your bust.

- Wear T-shirts that are slightly ruched in the middle. This will confuse the eye and draw the focus away from your tummy

- Shirts, blouses and dresses with slight V-necks are flattering.

- The best length for your tops (when worn with pants) is just below your hipbone.

- Long sleeves or dresses with sleeves help draw attention from your waist, shoulders, and arms.

- V-necks draw attention to your neck and bust and help create a vertical line

- Tops that drape over any curves work well.

- Choose tops that draw attention to your arms and away from your belly, such as ones with slight flares or a flit of embroidery

- Longer tops and jackets that skim the body can be worn with leggings or skinny jeans
- Wear bottoms just below your hipbone to help draw attention away from your midriff.
- Tailored jackets with a nice V shape at the top are very flattering.
- Make sure the jacket fits your shoulders perfectly, so choose the size for your shoulders and not your belly. If you can't close the jacket you can always use a scarf to fill the gap if you'd like.
- Patterns tend to look very good, as they flatter and help camouflage.
- Asymmetry in your tops helps create vertical lines that are slimming.
- Dark colors help camouflage the heavy areas.
- Layer your clothes with a long cardigan or a long sleeveless vest.
- Pants with a high rise help create a nice silhouette.
- Wear trousers and jeans with some stretch for extra comfort and a good fit.
- Choose skirts and pants with zippers at the sides.
- Structured pencil skirts, preferably at knee length, work well.

DON'T:

- Avoid dresses and belts that cinch the waist.
- Avoid tops that are sheer or made of thin materials. Choose ones with thicker textures, such as woven tops, since they don't cling so much.
- Stay away from skinny and straight-leg pants as they emphasize the hips. Choose slightly flared pants instead. These help balance wide shoulders and a heavy upper body.

- Avoid trousers and skirts that have zippers on the front as they add bulk to the front.

- Wear jeans that are tailored and either straight or slightly flared. Trouser jeans are ideal.

- Avoid skirts that have pleats starting above the belly, to avoid extra volume.

- Avoid big puffy jackets and tops.

- Stay away from shapeless garments that don't show any waist.

- Avoid horizontal patterns, pleats, and layers.

- Stay away from bulky trousers with lots of pockets.

- Tops with high necklines should be replaced with lighter tops underneath a layering piece instead.

- Stay away from tight, clingy tops and T-shirts.

- Avoid wearing everything in one solid color. Mix colors and textures or use several layers in different colors to create vertical lines instead.

PEAR

The aim of dressing for your body type is to achieve a nice hourglass shape, a flattering look that accentuates your strengths. Since your hips are a lot wider than your shoulders and you have a very good upper body, much of the emphasis in dressing is to draw attention to your upper body and waist and accentuate your shoulders and widen them. Because you tend to store weight on your thighs and your legs may be heavy, you will want to choose to dress in styles that will elongate your legs.

DO:

- Wear clothes that emphasize the upper body, that add to your shoulder and bust area and that make your hips look slimmer.

- Tops that accentuate shoulders, such as the current trendy off-shoulder blouses, are perfect.

- Always make sure that the shoulders are properly fitted

- Wear trousers that are not too tight or light. Boot-leg trousers and straight-leg pants are perfect.

- Wear tops with a catchy color or some nice detail such as big collars, breast pockets, or a pattern.

- Horizontal stripes help to widen your upper body to bring it more into balance with your hips, as do slim shoulder pads.

- Make sure your tops or jackets end either above or below the widest point of your hips.

- To emphasize your small waist, wear waist belts.

- Keep your tops in light colors, and make your trousers or skirt the darkest part of your outfit.

- Structured A-line coats, preferably knee length, with details on the top, such as lapels on shoulders, can be very flattering. The trench coat is ideal.

- A-line dresses and dresses with defined shoulders look particularly good on you.

- V-neckline tops help draw attention to your upper body.

- High boots can be very flattering for your legs, as are shoes with medium to chunky heels with a bit of height to further elongate your legs.

- Wearing a good bra that adds to or enhances your bust is recommended.

- Short jackets help break up your elongated torso, giving the illusion of longer legs.

DON'T:

- To minimize the lower half avoid pants or tights that narrow your legs. Flared pants can make your legs look thick, even bow-legged.

- Avoid skinny jeans (except when worn with tunics or A-line tops).

- Avoid short skirts and pencil or straight skirts.

- Stay away from tops with narrow shoulder lines.

- Pleats and pants with lots of detailing are a no-no.

- Shoes with ankle straps or kitten heels and other delicate footwear will shorten your legs.

RULER/RECTANGLE

Ruler is the most dominant body shape after the pear shape. This is one of the easier body types for dressing, and many models tend to have this body shape. A lot of clothes suit you and fit you well, although those who are taller may have trouble finding clothes that fit properly.

You will want to create more curves and can do this by defining your waist as well as wearing clothes that help create curves on the top or the bottom. A straight look is also flattering by surrendering the waistline altogether.

DO:

- Wear clothes that create curves by focusing on the upper and lower part of your body.
- Cinch your waist to exaggerate curves by wearing belts.
- Wear flared skirts with fitted belted waistbands.
- Knee-length pencil skirts that taper in at the sides will add curves and look good.
- A-line skirts work really well for this body type.
- Tight pants and slightly flared trousers all look great on you. Low- to mid-waisted pants are usually best.
- Blouses can look really good if they are tucked in.
- Use strong colors to help define your body.
- Wear coats and jackets that emphasize the waist or that are belted at the waist.
- Jackets that are slightly padded at the shoulders are flattering.
- Medium to high necklines work well, especially if you have a small bust and long neck.
- To create the illusion of a larger bust, choose tops with pockets, ruching, pleating, or other front details. Halter necklines are also flattering.

- If you are long waisted, chunky belts can look really good.
- Dresses or tops with embellishment at the bust, or with frills and ruffles at the top, will add some volume to make your chest look bigger.
- Shift dresses, empire-line dresses, and dropped-waist dresses all look good.
- Skinny jeans, miniskirts and bright tights that show off your great legs and add more shape to a straight body are recommended.
- Three-quarter sleeves are flattering
- A bra that adds a cup size will help balance your angular feature as well.

DON'T:

- Avoid boyish/manly and shapeless clothes.
- Baggy jeans, flared pants, and track clothes will make you look like "one of the boys."
- For working out, wear feminine track clothes that accentuate your waist but are not too snug on the top and bottom halves.
- Avoid belts if you have no waist at all.
- If you want to add curves then avoid straight dresses.

INVERTED TRIANGLE

This is quite a desirable shape, as many clothes look good on you. To achieve an ideal hourglass body shape you will want to draw attention away from your big upper chest and broad shoulders, and at the same time bring the focus to your slim lower body and legs, which are often lean with this body type.

DO:

- Keep your attention on the waist and hip area by wearing clothes that are flared on the bottom but snug on the top.
- Strapless tops and dresses with sleeves are perfect.
- Flared pants and pleated skirts are flattering.
- Wear tops with vertical lines, such as vertical stripes and vertical prints.
- Wear tops with open necklines and collars, like halters, V-necklines, and scoop necklines.
- Wear soft feminine textures to soften the shoulder line.
- Wear darker colors on top.
- Wear jackets that are well-structured at the shoulder, and wear them open and unbuttoned, to create a vertical line.
- Single-breasted tailored jackets help eliminate extra width on top.
- Wear A-lines or full skirts to create more width and overall balance.
- Horizontal stripes on skirts will make the lower body wider and create balance
- Full or boot-leg pants as well as culottes work well
- Pockets or embellishments on trousers and skirts are flattering.
- Use bold textures on the lower body to create more bulk.

DON'T:

- Avoid skinny pants and too-tight skirts.

- Avoid dresses or tops with ruffles and flounces, or that are off-the-shoulder, as they will make you look top heavy.

- Avoid shoulder pads or anything that accentuates the shoulders.

- Stay away from dresses or tops with bateau necklines.

- Keep away from horizontal prints, big bold patterns and graphics on top, as they have a widening effect.

- Avoid oversized collars and lapels on jackets.

- If you must wear chunky knits, choose dark solid colors.

- Avoid tapered skirts.

The guidelines listed here are for general guidance only, as everyone is different. Many women are a mix of two body types and don't necessarily fall into one category or another. In that case, try incorporating tips for each body type and see what looks best on you. When you fall between two types, compare the type you seem closest to and pick styles that lean toward that. Ultimately, you will know what feels good and what flatters you the most. After all, there is no right or wrong way to dress. Your comfort and your confidence are what matter most.

"SELF-CONFIDENCE IS THE BEST OUTFIT. ROCK IT AND OWN IT."

—RANI ST. PUCCHI

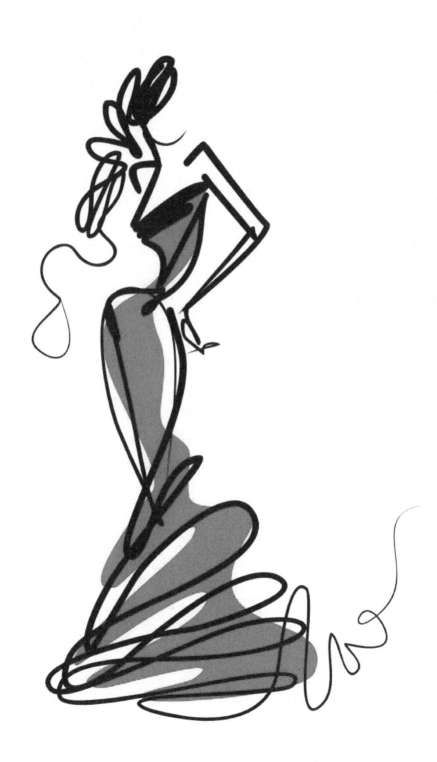

CHAPTER THREE

Aside from the five body types we discussed in previous chapters, there are other attributes that are worth looking at.

If you are . . .

SHORT AND THIN

- Avoid clothes with too much volume, full-length coats, and wide maxi dresses, as they will be too overpowering.

- Select simple and fitted clothes that form long vertical lines.

- Single colors and vertical stripes will make you look taller.

- Cropped jackets, shorts, mini dresses, and skirts help keep your petite frame in perfect proportion.

- Choose curved silhouettes to look wider.

- Elongate your legs by wearing high heels.

SHORT AND HEAVY

- Choose colors and patterns wisely.

- Solid, dark colors, such as navy, black, dark brown, and deep purple, minimize curves, handles, or bulges you wish to hide.

- Stay away from voluminous and elaborate dresses, as these styles make you look shorter and smaller.

- Stay away from oversized floral and horizontal prints, as these only make you look wider.

- Stay away from wide belts and cummerbunds, which make you appear shorter.

TALL AND THIN

- You can choose to wear almost any style of clothes, from A-line to full skirts and flared bottoms.

- To accentuate your long body and appear even taller, wear straight, vertical designs and fitted dresses.

- To appear shorter, opt for a two-piece ensemble instead.

- A cropped top or a ruffled over-blouse can be very flattering.

- Flared skirts add grace to your height and straight skirts exaggerate it.

- Tiny prints, delicate jewelry, and sheer fabric will exaggerate your height.

- Wide belts and cummerbunds help make you look shorter.

TALL AND HEAVY

- A dress or blouse with an off-the-shoulder neckline will make your upper body more in proportion to your lower half.

- An A-line silhouette that is fitted at the shoulders and flares away from the bodice helps create a clean, flowing line. This camouflages the larger hips by creating a slight triangle to the lower half of the body.

- An empire style that is fitted and cinched under the bust and flows freely will help disguise your heaviness.

SHORT-WAISTED AND TALL

- Wear dresses that have seams a few inches below the natural waistline.

- Wear tops that reach below the natural waistline or that are tucked out to elongate the waist.

- Wear long jackets.

- Wear low-waisted skirts and pants.

- Wear non-contrasting belts.

SHORT-WAISTED AND SHORT

- Select dresses that have vertical seams from under the bust, as they will elongate your figure.

- Clothes that have no specific waistline are also perfect.

- Keep to one color rather than contrasts.

- If you wear a belt then it should be monotone or at least match your top, not your bottom.

- Fitted sleeves help give an illusion of longer arms and a longer waistline.

LONG-WAISTED

- To shorten the bodice, select styles with a strong horizontal emphasis, like yokes, wide waistlines, extended shoulders, or bateau necklines.

- Wear short to medium-length tops and jackets.
- A-lines with moderately flared skirts are also appropriate.
- Classic wide pants look great on you.
- Avoid tight, tapered skirts and pants.
- Avoid skirts and trousers with a dropped waistband.
- Stay away from any prints or adornments that hit at hip level.
- Don't blouson your tops.
- Avoid cropped pants.
- Wear a medium to wide belt that is not the same color as your top. A contrasting belt is better.
- Short sleeves or even elbow-length sleeves work best for this body type.

SMALL BUST

- To create a little drama and enhance your bustline select styles with lots of detail in the bust area. Ruffled, flared necklines are also perfect.
- A padded bra always helps.
- Looser, relaxed tops are better than a stretch bodysuit.
- If your hips are bigger than your bust, try adding straight elements in your wardrobe, such as a straight skirt, to balance your silhouette.
- Full sleeves with ruffles and puffed (or Gibson) sleeves are all good options and help add fullness to the bodice area.

FULL BUST

- To draw your attention away from the bust wear A-line dresses, or dresses with long bodices and a full skirt. These will make your bust look slender.

- Never sacrifice your waist. Stylishly belting your dress will help create a beautiful head-to-toe hourglass.

- If your bust is bigger than your hips, wear a skirt that flares from the hips to create a nice balance.

- If your bust is the same size as your hips and you have a nice waistline then try a straight silhouette to make the most of your beautiful figure.

- Fitted sleeves help make you look slender, as do dolman and kimono sleeves.

SHORT LEGS

- High-waisted dresses and skirts are recommended.

- High-waisted jeans and pants look good, as they make your legs blend in with your upper body.

- Skirts that end right at the knee can give the appearance of elongated legs.

- Avoid skirts or dresses that go past the knee, as they will make your legs look short and chubby.

SLENDER/PETITE

- If you're small boned and under 5 foot 4 wear clothes that don't overwhelm your delicate frame.

- Wear dresses and tops that are strapless, as they draw the eye upward.

- Opt for clothes with a close, body-hugging fit, and keep accessories to a minimum.

- Open heels will lengthen legs.

- Avoid too many competing elements in any one single outfit.

CURVY/PETITE

- Curves can look exaggerated on smaller frames, so the trick is in how you play with proportion.
- Wear dresses that are fitted on top and flow from the hips to create balance.
- Wear blouses that are soft and flowing.
- Avoid overly detailed jeans, pants, and skirts.
- Cropped jeans should only be worn with high heels.

FULL-FIGURED

- Wear dresses with an empire waist or long inverted pleats.
- Vertical lines in print are slenderizing.
- Always show a little skin at the neck and décolletage by wearing open necklines.
- Tops with V-necklines are great.
- Keep shapes simple and avoid ruffles and too much embellishment.

"Every day is a and the world is

fashion show
the runway."

—*Coco Chanel*

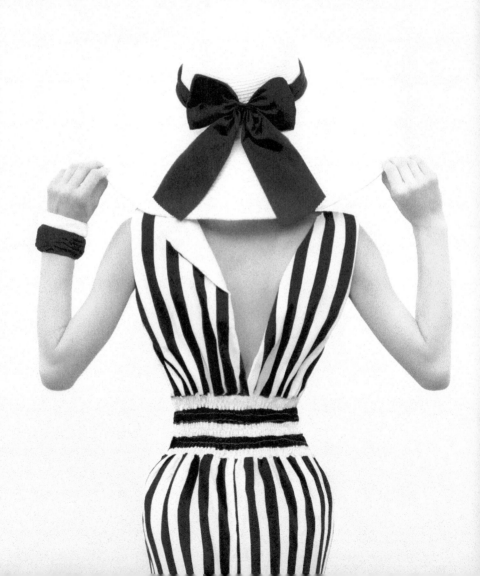

CHAPTER FOUR

Have your hot pants reached their expiration date? Or that short, short black skirt that you loved so much and hung onto for decades, is it time to let it go?

Dressing for your age is not what it used to be. Women today are extremely active and mindful of their looks and their bodies. It used to be that minis were off the table after a certain age and a woman over 50 was told to watch those sleeveless tops and plunging necklines. Not so today.

Strict dictums about what to wear and when to wear it have no place in the times we live in. Just like a Botoxed wrinkle fades in the blink of an eye, so have the rules been tossed aside. Yes, your body changes as you age, but that does not mean that you should give up a youthful lifestyle and way of dressing.

As you age, your taste, your budget, and your lifestyle change as well. Dressing your age is really about making sure your clothes reflect who you are now and how confident they make you feel. You can embrace sexy and keep your edge as long as it's done tastefully.

IN YOUR 20s

You want to make sure you never look matronly. Thick, nude pantyhose and frumpy skirts and oversized shirts and tops are off the table. Be playful. Wear pretty, girlie dresses and edgy ensembles, show some leg, and do it now, while you can, so there are no regrets. Take chances and experiment with pairing unusual silhouettes, and rock that jewelry and those necklaces and cuffs.

You can be ladylike when you feel like it; Bohemian, all-American, or glamorous when you fancy. You can dress as the girl next door. Your style can be sultry, or you can be the goddess . . . Take your pick. Because you can. And because anything goes when you're a 20-something.

IN YOUR 30s

Your taste inches upward, and you learn to start investing in timeless pieces, such as a smart blazer or a glamorous, seductive, and elegant black dress that will never go out of style.

You get serious about fit, and you still mix it up, but now you're looking to be more elegant.

You embrace sexy because you have the confidence and the authority to pull it off.

IN YOUR 40s

You find yourself becoming more practical. You shop strategically and invest in a few luxury items, such as a designer coat, an embellished evening dress, or a well-tailored suit.

You keep your edge by combining a few classic pieces, such as a leather blazer, a croc bag, or a pair of embellished heels. You want to look classic and smart.

You steer clear of fussy clothes, such as bows and ruffles, and girlie prints and matronly, shapeless suits.

On occasions when you find yourself wanting to wear slim dresses and skirts and get a more defined waist you opt to wear shapewear under your clothes.

You've kept yourself in great shape and you feel confident in almost anything, slinky sexy gowns included.

IN YOUR 50S

You're enjoying life to the fullest, and you feel there is still a lot of fun to be had. After all, 50 is the new 40, and you're full of ideas and plans and can't wait to explore the next 50 years!

You dress to express your truth. You are decisive. You have defined your look. Now it's all about fit and confidence.

You play with colors that are flattering to your skin and hair color and choose shades that work best for you.

You dress for impact, by coordinating pieces that layer and travel well.

You splurge on statement pieces, such as a signature cuff, a chunky necklace, a cashmere hoodie, a luxury watch.

IN YOUR 60S AND BEYOND

In your 60s your aim is to look young and hip but still age appropriate. Your elegance becomes you. You go for guilty pleasures and feel free to splurge—just because you deserve it. You're too self-assured to invest in trendy pieces that may be here today but gone tomorrow.

You still go for classic, timeless clothing, such as trim trousers and suits, jackets, and dresses that are current.

You know when it's appropriate to show your legs and your arms, and you keep them toned. You cover when you have to, with a chic wrap, and add a little shine that flatters your skin with a jacket that has a rich fur or a brocade trim.

You add color to your everyday wardrobe and have fun dressing and show it in your clothes. Your dresses drape in all the right places and you like classic, versatile garments that fit perfectly.

You are inspired to look your best and most elegant, and you have cultivated your own strong fashion style that is uniquely yours. Your personality has evolved over the years, and you are totally comfortable in your skin. There is nothing you need to prove to anyone. It's all about you now.

> "You can be gorgeous at *thirty*, charming at forty, and irresistible for the *rest of your life*."
>
> —Coco Chanel

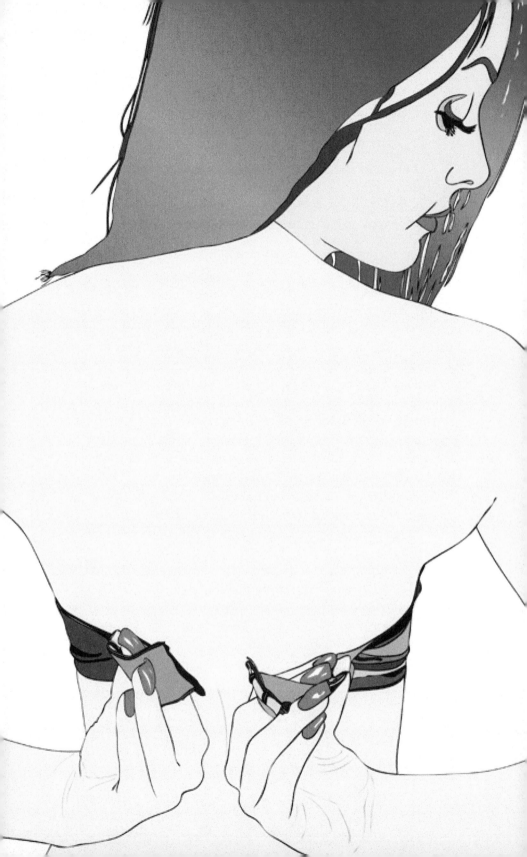

CHAPTER FIVE

"Without proper foundations there can be no fashion."
—Christian Dior

HAVING A FIT?

Bras are notoriously hard to shop for and never seem to fit right. Between learning about correct band sizes and cup sizes, the various misconceptions that exist around bras and finding a bra that fits can be mind-blowing.

According to a leading bra manufacturer, 80 percent of women today wear the wrong size bra. It's mainly because they never bother to get professionally measured and instead base their choice of bra size on common assumptions of what an A-cup or a D-cup supposedly looks like:

A = small
B = average
C = medium
D = large
DD or anything over that = really large

Needless to say, these assumptions are entirely incorrect. Your cup size is not about the size of your breasts, but in fact is an indicator of the difference between your band size (which is the circumference of your back, just below your breasts) and the circumference of your breasts. Therefore, every inch difference means that you have to go up or down one size. The relationship between band and cup size can be utterly confusing, and it is best left to the experts in the lingerie department to help you determine your true size.

Be prepared to try on as many different bras as possible until you find your favorite. Different brands fit differently even though they may indicate the same size, as do different styles and size combinations. Beware of international sizing as well, as they do not necessarily correspond to what you are used to.

When you wear band sizes that are either too small or too big your bra can't do its job—which is to make your clothes look good!

Little things mean a lot indeed, so don't skimp. After all, your carefully considered clothes will never look right without the proper underpinnings. Start with your bras, and take the time to find the shapes you need in the perfect size for you. You can find assistance from a professional in the lingerie department to officially size you up.

SOLUTIONS TO COMMON BRA ISSUES

BIG-CHESTED

Anyone with a D-cup upward must realize the importance of a well-fitted bra. Make sure it is made in a smooth fabric rather than of lace and that there is an underwire, since this will help push the breasts forward as well as upward. Wearing a loose, ill-fitting bra can cause back problems.

SMALL-CHESTED

Make sure the gore (the part between the cups in front) lies against your chest as opposed to floating between them. If not, then a padded bra might help, but make sure it's not *so* heavily padded as to look fake and allow others to see the fraud in your cleavage.

FLAT-CHESTED

If you are so flat-chested that your breasts generally go in different directions, leaving a raised flat blank space in the center, you need to fill the underneath section to bring your breasts together in the middle.

SAGGY BOOBS

The ultimate bra to lift your bust is called the *balcony*. This design lovingly cups, ups, and separates your breasts to provide the perfect shape akin to a cosmetic lift, allowing you to wear and look great in clothes.

FLABBY BACK

Most of us can relate to having a fat back. You need a wide strap that will distribute the pulling power over a wider area, thus reducing the flesh-digging capabilities.

BACK OF YOUR BRA RIDES UP

If the back of your bra rides up*:*
   Try tightening the hook or loosening the straps. If that doesn't work then go down a size. Make sure your bra lies flat against your back without riding up or sitting too low. It's fine if the band digs into your skin a tiny bit, since it should be tight, but it should never feel restricting or painful.

ROLLS OF FLESH ABOVE BACK STRAP

If there *are rolls of flesh above back straps:*
   Breast tissue spilling out on the sides and above the straps means the band (as opposed to the cup) size may be too small or there is a shape mismatch.

STRAPS CONSTANTLY FALLING DOWN

If your straps fall down cons*tantly:*

Adjust the bra straps and make sure they are at the correct length. The straps should be tight enough to stay on your shoulders without digging into the skin. If adjusting the straps doesn't work then the slope of your shoulders could be the problem. In this case a T-back shape may work best.

WRINKLY BRA CUPS

If the bra cups are wrinkly:

Try getting into the bra this way: lean over and let your breasts "fall" into the cups. If that doesn't fix the creasing, you may need to go down one band size.

SPILLING OUT OF YOUR BRA

If you're spilling out of your bra*:*

If you're bursting out at the sides or over the top of the cups, you may need a larger cup size or a shape with more coverage on the sides and top. The cups should lie flat against your breasts without gaping at the top or causing a spillover.

If a bra alone does not do the trick and you need more support then do consider a corset in addition to the bra. A corset can work magic. It supports and lets you wear what you want without worrying about bulges, bust support, waistline, or even posture—although in sweltering heat it can be just one more layer to make you sweat.

YOUR LOWER BODY

Get a little waist management and avoid visible panty lines to smooth the lower half of your body and torso. Flabby stomach, saggy hips, cellulite behind, and big thighs can all be corrected by wearing specialty panties that maximize or minimize and lift the butt.

A too-tight waistband can cause flab to flip from underneath and create rolls, while a G-string and bikini briefs can be the worst enemy of a sagging butt as they offer no support whatsoever. Neither do the satin and lace cami-panties work if you have big thighs and a saggy behind. Instead invest in hips and thigh panties with extra thick Lycra that will hold in and redistribute the flesh to give you a slim and thin appearance. The ultimate solution is a pair of contouring panties, such as the Spanx Power Panties, which afford a finish that is smooth and allows clothes to slide on with confidence.

The right shapewear that is soft but supportive can help smooth you out and distribute fat evenly while at the same time giving definition to areas like the bust and thighs. It's the best solution for any clothing that is form-fitting.

Tights, girdles, body-shapers, and all-in-ones are readily available today for the sole purpose of improving our shape. The resulting effect is instant gratification, minimizing hours spent sweating at the gym and giving us permission to consume calories guilt-free!

So it bears mentioning that you can't neglect the lingerie fundamentals, since they really can make or break your look. Get the right fit and your clothes will look like a million bucks.

Go beyond the basics and get the underwear right. You can change how your clothes fit instantly by incorporating the correct underpinnings. Just because these are worn underneath, women think, *"Who cares? No one is going to see it."* Not so.

Most women think that the underwear has to be either sexy *or* supporting—you *can* get underwear that serves both functions. Likewise, if you're having a crisis of confidence, an easy way to feel desirable again is to invest in sexy and supportive bras and underwear. And for those women who are going through menopause, it helps to get the support in all areas that have given in to gravity.

"Brevity is the soul of lingerie."

—*Dorothy Parker*

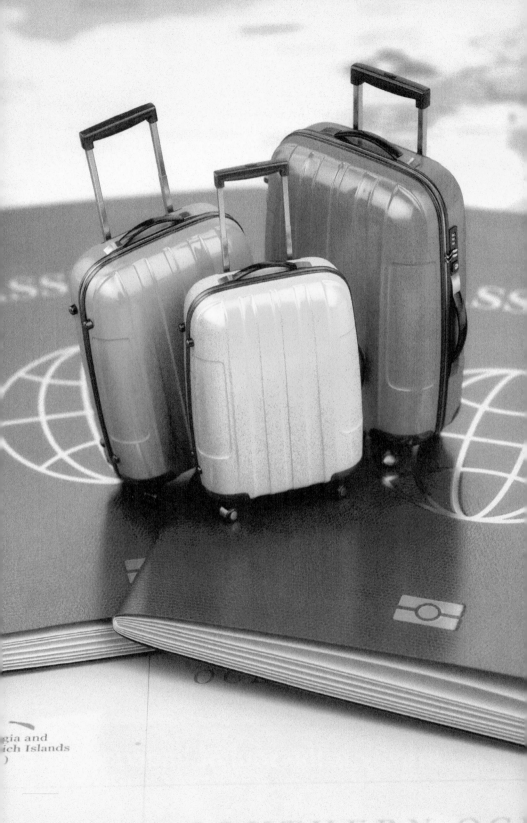

CHAPTER SIX

Ask any adventure virtuoso, backpacker, or business traveler what is the most time-consuming (and confusing) part of planning for a trip, and invariably they will all say packing.

Having a good holiday lies in the preparation. Checking the weather then arriving to a place where the temperature turned unexpectedly and not being prepared can be one of the most frustrating things.

OH, THE PLACES YOU'LL GO, BUT WHAT TO WEAR?

There is nothing worse than traveling to a country and not bringing the right clothes or your favorite products because you didn't think there was enough room in your suitcase. Anything can happen on a foreign journey. The success of your trip is in planning so you're prepared to face any situation. Thinking that you can purchase what you didn't pack, only to be disappointed because they had never heard of the brand you use, can be outright frustrating.

What about over packing "just in case" you need something, and then realizing that half the clothes you took with you were not even touched? Besides, you had to haul all that weight and even pay the airlines for excess baggage because of all the other stuff you shopped for.

Making sure that your return will be just as happy based on how good you look in those holiday photos is just as important. After all, you want to capture beautiful memories as keepsakes to show your family as well as revisit them in the future. And don't forget that you want to show off to all your social media "friends" what a fabulous time you had.

You want to look great, naturally poised, and fabulous so you can be the envy of everyone. Unless you're perfect, you cannot leave your photo appearance to chance. So you need some careful planning.

Perhaps you're one of those seasoned travelers and a gifted packer, in the sense that you know exactly what to take and effortlessly pop them in those suitcases. You know exactly what will be required: the right outfits, shoes, underwear, tampons, shampoo, sun lotion, and anything and everything else. You're going with the assumption that all countries are third world and unable to provide for your daily necessities. You also remember to include an empty bag to bring back all the stuff you'll be shopping for there. If so, then good for you!

Unfortunately for most of us, even though we've traveled often enough, this process can be grueling, and without fail we forget to bring something or other. Equally as draining as jet lag and having to stand in long lines at check-in is that late-night moment when you face the empty suitcase and wonder what on earth should you fill it with.

So, how can you get this process down to a science so you don't have any regrets and spoil your trip wishing, even blaming someone else for your choices? How much to bring?

PLANNING FOR THE TRIP

Several days before the trip, check the weather to determine what you will need. List all the items you will need, and keep the list where you can see it often. Each time you remember something, add it to the list. The list should be divided into: clothes, shoes, undergarments, workout clothes (if needed), swimwear, nightclothes, toiletries, camera items, and any other necessities that are part of your daily regiment.

WHAT TO PACK

FOR A BUSINESS TRIP

Classics and neutrals work best. A black pantsuit, a well-tailored herringbone sheath, a classic trench, a white shirt, and a sleek jacket are some basic pieces that will keep you looking sharp. Pack a couple of scarves to add color and some jewelry to dress up your outfit for evenings out.

FOR A SHORT OVERNIGHT TRIP

You need one pair of bottoms with two interchangeable tops; make one dressy and the other casual. Add a cardigan, sweater, or jacket.

FOR A LONG WEEKEND

Think in terms of mix-and-match pieces. Three tops, two bottoms, and one dress will give you more than six different outfits. Add a pair of yoga pants that can double as pajamas. And a swimsuit.

FOR A LONGER TRIP OF A WEEK OR MORE

Get six days right. Plot them from head to toe. Add to the mix some camisoles and underpinnings and at least two jackets and a couple of scarves. Now you're comfortably prepared for twelve to sixteen outfits that can be interchangeable by rotating the tops and bottoms, switching camisoles, and changing accessories. Add to the mix two yoga pants and a swimsuit.

TRAVELING TO TROPICAL DESTINATIONS

If you're departing in drifts and arriving in the tropics then make sure to pack a beach bag that can fit your sunscreen, towel, and a book. The bag should be large enough but not so big that you cannot use it as a purse as well. Pack two sun hats: a structured straw hat, and a fold-up cotton one to keep in your bag so you'll always be protected. Pack an umbrella, too, just in case.

Layer your clothing. Make a T your base layer and have a lightweight shirt you can throw over, along with espadrilles or open toed flats for easy walking.

Always pack a chameleon item or two that can be worn in multiple ways, such as a tunic dress that you can slip over a bathing suit, which can also be dressed up for an evening out when paired with the right sandals and earrings. A lightweight sweater or cardigan can be draped over your sexy camisole for the evening.

PACKING YOUR SHOES

Footwear is probably the hardest part to get right. Your shoes need to work extra hard, but since they take up much more room and are some of the heaviest items to pack, you don't want to take too many. You will want two pairs, one dressy and one casual, in colors that are interchangeable and match your wardrobe best. Pack a pair of sneakers, too, just in case.

Make sure you do not take new pairs of shoes that have not been broken in, as you run the risk of getting blisters from too much walking. Test-walk in your shoes again and again before packing. Make sure they are secure and stable on the feet and provide support as well as have soles that have traction. There is nothing worse than sore feet.

PACKING PURSES AND BAGS

Avoid packing too many purses and bags. An ideal bag is one that has a shorter handle (for evenings) plus a longer cross-body *wide strap* (for daytime touring). After several hours of walking, your shoulders can hurt if your bag is too heavy. The wide strap is a must for the cross-body to be comfortable on the shoulder.

TRAVELING WITH SMALL CHILDREN AND BABIES

When you're traveling with little children it gets a little more complicated. You want to think about practicality as well as comfort and style. Pack colors that won't show dirt and grime, and fabrics that can be chucked into a washing machine. You will have to deal with sticky fingers and flying drinks, so you don't want to have to worry about your whites and neutrals, and velvets and silks.

HOW TO PACK YOUR SUITCASE

The easiest trick to avoiding wrinkles when packing is to fold the garment in a plastic bag or use layers of tissue between the folds. It's best to pack all the lightweight and smaller stuff first. The typical way most of us have been taught to pack is to put the heavy stuff at the bottom so it doesn't squash our clothes.

In fact the best way is the reverse, especially when you're going on a long trip. The heavier clothes on top act as a press and keep the items underneath from wriggling around and getting creased. You also have more nooks and crannies in which to stuff little bits and pieces and small items that can be rolled into tiny bundles and placed in the grooves at the bottom.

OVERPACKING

Now that your suitcase is packed you test the weight and find out it's really not that heavy and there's still some room. You decide that you can sneak in a hand luggage and a few more pairs of shoes and clothes. Stop! Beware of packing too much. If you find your suitcase is too heavy for you to carry by yourself, then it's time to stop adding more to it.

Dragging heavy, over packed luggage can be a killjoy on your journey. You may find yourself in countries and places where your big and heavy suitcases barely fit the tiny elevators in your hotel, or worse still that you have to haul them up narrow and winding marble staircases that are steep and never-ending!

Imagine the regret. You fell victim to the "just in case" mentality, and brought clothing and shoes that were never even unpacked, let alone worn. Moreover you decided to bring multiples of everything . . . Just in case!

Remember that no one is going to notice if you wore the same outfit every third day, or that you had the same cardigan every day. The trick is to give your clothes a different spin by letting your accessories add variety. Jewelry, scarves and belts can easily make the same clothing look different and interesting.

Make sure that before you pack, you try everything on, in all the variations and combinations you can think of. This is the wardrobe you will be living in, so it must work well and look good for where you're heading. Ditch anything that is not comfortable or you're not too sure you will need.

An experienced traveler never packs an outfit that she hasn't rehearsed. That way she is certain that her coat fits well over her dress, and her shoes are comfortable, that she has the right accessories and everything works well together.

When in doubt take snapshots of the outfits in the combinations you have planned and rehearsed. That way it will be a no-brainer and save you angst and time rather than second-guessing what to wear. The pictures will remind you of the choices you had made and help you stick to your original plan.

YOUR CARRY-ON BAG

For the long-haul flight, your carry on is your best friend. Carry with you anything that is essential, and don't depend on your luggage getting there. Make sure you pack in it all you need to stay comfortable on the flight.

Think of your airplane seat as your bedroom and think of the essentials that will keep you cozy and comfortable. Warm socks? A pill? Carrying with you items such as a scarf, socks, and a clear plastic bag filled with your miniature toiletries like toothpaste, a toothbrush, moisturizer, lip balm, refreshing eye drops, etc. will help your journey be more pleasurable. Wear layers and make comfort your priority, because the trip can be long and it can get really cold.

Last but not least: Upon your return from your trip, immediately make a list of things you had forgotten to take. Add them to the original list of essentials you need to pack every time you travel. Tape the list to the inside of your suitcase as a reminder so that your future travels will be smooth and effortless.

"Twenty years from now you will be more disappointed by the things you didn't do than by the ones you did do. So throw off the bowlines, sail away from the safe harbor. Catch the trade winds in your sails. Explore. Dream. Discover."

—*Mark Twain*

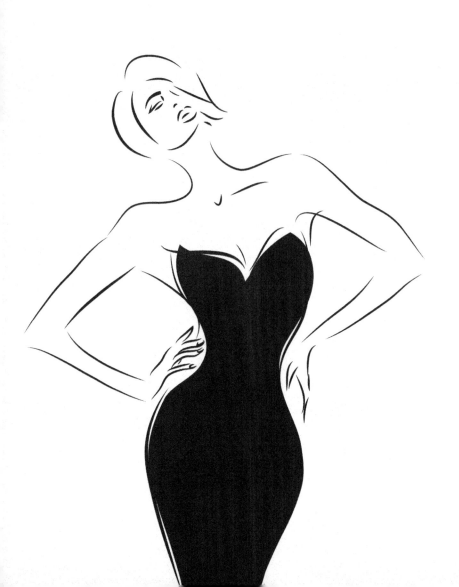

CHAPTER SEVEN

Any color, as long as it's black.
—*Henry Ford*

I f you could have only one dress in your wardrobe, wouldn't you make it a black one?

Black is uniquely powerful, mysterious, sophisticated, and seductive. Designers all over the world agree that black is the most slimming color in the spectrum.

Throughout history we have seen how the black dress has evolved. Women wore black for many reasons apart from mourning. It was a fashionable color for many European aristocrats, especially in the sixteenth century. Its popularity faded with the rise of French power in the seventeenth century but came back again strong in the nineteenth century and has not left us since.

Black has always played an important role in art as well. *Elegant* black is how artists and poets have referred with reverence to this color. *Portrait of Madame X* (1884) painted by John Singer Sargent caused a scandal in Parisian society. It depicts Madame Virginie Gautreau posing in an ultra-glamorous black dress. At the time, her pose was considered sexually suggestive. As originally exhibited, one strap of Gautreau's gown had fallen down her right shoulder, suggesting the possibility of further revelation; "One more struggle," wrote a critic in Le Figaro, "and the lady will be free." Ever since then, the diabolical black dress has been associated with that femme fatale image.

In Anna Karenina, Tolstoy hinted that his heroine was a sexual being, soon to be adulterous, and therefore doomed. He dressed his heroine in a "black, low-cut velvet gown, showing her full throat and shoulders, which looked as though carved in old ivory, and her rounded arms, with tiny, slender wrists."

The "little black dress" was actually born sometime in the early 1900s and eventually became the most fashionable color during World War I, because so many Europeans were in mourning.

So the belief that Coco Chanel invented the little black dress in the 1920s is not entirely accurate. Although with *American Vogue* showcasing her creation in their 1926 issue, her version of the style became extremely influential among the fashionable and the elite.

Why a black dress, you ask? Because black is glamorous, seductive, practical, chic, versatile, classic, elegant, powerful, and modern.

Need I say more?

Oh, yes, and black never goes out of style.

"Worldly, elegant, plainly alluring—indispensable."

—*British Vogue on black, September 1957*

There are as many shades of black as there are shades of gray. It would not be inaccurate to say that there are at least fifty shades of black. Depending on the fabric, the dye can take on variations of hues that range from pitch black to a hint of gray, orange, blue, violet, green, or yellow tones. Likewise, the black in velvet may be darker than the black in silk or cotton.

If you had one classic black dress in your wardrobe you could dress it up or down in numerous ways. A simple black sheath can become sensational when worn under a brocade or velvet jacket. A chunky necklace can immediately transport the same dress to one that is sexy and vibrant that will turn heads over a candlelit dinner. A jeweled belt can take the dress from day to evening.

When it comes to fashion, we're nocturnal creatures, and often times we may not have the budget to splurge on an evening outfit every season. While it may be tempting to run out and buy a new dress each time another invite arrives, the best approach is to have a mix-and-match evening wardrobe with the little black dress as the central focus.

ONE DRESS, UMPTEEN WAYS TO WEAR IT

Be creative with your little black dress by dressing it up with one of the variations listed below:

- Cropped jacket in velvet, brocade, or soft luxurious leather
- A short or long jacket
- A velvet, silk, or cashmere stole
- Long earrings
- Necklace: chunky or one with a pendant
- A multi-strand choker
- Layers and layers of pearls
- One enormous cuff bracelet
- An oversized pin on the shoulder
- An heirloom jeweled hairpin
- Jeweled belt or one with a decorative buckle
- Metallic sandals
- Evening pumps

- Glittery evening bag
- Evening clutch
- Fox (or faux) shrug

If you have these items you can create a variety of different looks with the one little black dress you own, looks that will be unique so that each time an opportunity comes your way to attend a special occasion or an evening out your attire will look fresh and new.

The little black dress is the ultimate chameleon, the one piece of clothing that is worth your investment.

"Elegance does not consist of putting on a new dress."

—*Coco Chanel*

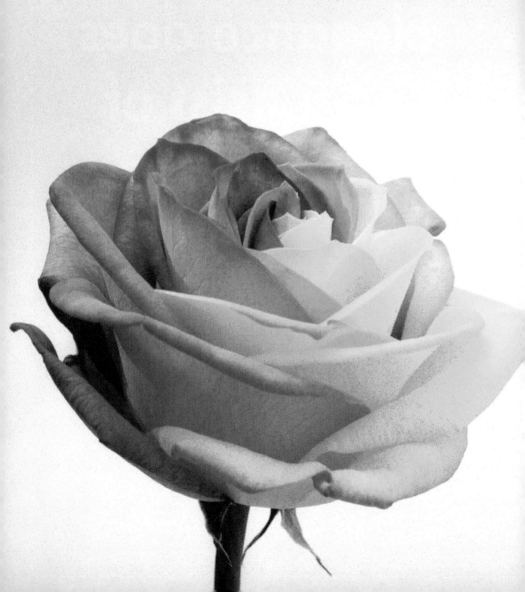

CHAPTER EIGHT

COLOR

"Let me, O let me bathe my
soul in colors; let me swallow the
sunset and drink the rainbow."

— *Kahlil Gibran*

FEELING DEPRESSED? UNMOTIVATED TO GET READY IN THE MORNING?

The cure lies in your wardrobe.

It's fascinating how wearing the right colors can boost your confidence and give you that spring in your step. Why fit in with the crowd when you can stand out as an individual?

Those who understand color and know what colors look great on them look more vibrant, self-assured, confident, and interesting. They feel more in control, more attractive, and more elegant. Wearing the right color can make you look slimmer, healthier, shorter, or taller.

It's a well-known fact that color can influence your mood. Picking colors to wear each morning based on how you're feeling, happy or sad, is an unconscious choice we all tend to make. If you're happy you will normally choose something colorful to wear, and if you're a little sad or depressed you tend to gravitate toward dull colors or even all black.

However, if you are mindful and determined to change your mood, it can be done with no effort at all. Rather than choosing colors to match your mood, go for a color that will enforce the mood you wish to be in. It's very hard to keep feeling sad or depressed when you are wearing a bright color.

THE PSYCHOLOGY OF COLOR

Wearing clothes in certain colors can affect you differently. Let's look at some of these colors and the moods they can invoke.

Violet (Purple/Indigo): Royalty, wealth, prosperity, sophistication, respect, ambition, creativity, success, mystery, spirituality, healing, calmness, wisdom. Violet is a great protective color as it connects with our intuition and psychic abilities and enhances transformation. This is a good color to wear on days when you need to tap into creativity and success. It lends an air of mystery, wisdom, and respect and stimulates the brain activity used in problem-solving.

Wear this to feel calm and invoke creativity.

Blue: Calmness, serenity, care, cooperation, power, reliability, loyalty, dignity, harmony, balance, compassion, security. Blue can stimulate productivity and helps bring focus on the task at hand as well as boost performance. It is associated with steadfastness, dependability, wisdom, and loyalty.

This is a good color when you want to feel calm and be more intuitive.

Green: Comfort, compassion, empathy, health, progress, efficiency, prosperity, generosity, freedom, fertility, faith, adventure. Green is a calming color that's very pleasing to the senses and is a traditional color of peace and harmony. The color green allows us to let go of old pain and grudges and creates space for the acceptance of others and ourselves. It promotes inner tranquility and invites others to trust more.

Use this color to ease your anxiety and feel more relaxed.

Yellow: Happiness, optimism, warmth, friendship, intelligence, innovation, inspiration, power, alertness. The color yellow helps boost our confidence and our outlook on life with positivity and provides direction and determination when needed. It is the color of the sun, associated with laughter, happiness, and optimism, and it helps speed up our metabolisms as well as bring out creative ideas. It is known as the happiest color in the color spectrum.

Yellow is great to wear on days when you want to feel more optimistic, mentally stimulated and creative.

Orange: Communication, determination, independence, motivation, generosity, domination, competence, change, charisma. The color orange is the most flamboyant color on the planet. It excites the brain and boosts enthusiasm and ambition, and it is associated with a new dawn in attitude. It brings joy as well as stabilizes emotions.

Wear orange when you want to socialize and stimulate activity and conversation.

Red: Alertness, charm, aggression, courage, domination, eccentricity, energy, rebellion, sensuality, passion, desire, luck. The color red helps energize and rejuvenate us when we are tired, and is associated with movement and excitement. It can be a powerful manifesting color and gives us courage for a new beginning. Red symbolizes love and giving.

Wear red when you wish to tap into your courage and have lots of energy and confidence.

Pink: Romance, love, calmness, peace, happiness. Pink is the most calming of all colors and is the true color of love. It invokes gentle feelings and a soothing demeanor, and brings peace and calm to the environment.

Wear pink to feel more loving and at peace with others.

Brown: Stability, harmony, reliability, friendship. Brown is the color of the earth itself. It is associated with all things natural, harmonious, and organic.

Wear brown when you want to feel stable and wholesome.

Black: Power, authority, intelligence, stability, strength. Black is a somber color often associated with evil as well as with death and grieving in the Western culture. The color black is considered a sophisticated and slimming color to wear, although you can easily overwhelm people with too much black.

Use Black to feel powerful, authoritative, or mysterious.

White: Innocence, emptiness, peace, sterility, purity, cleanliness, spaciousness, neutrality. The color white is also used as a color of death or mourning in certain religions.

Wear white for more mental clarity.

Gold/Silver: Gold implies wealth, glamour, wisdom, and love, while silver evokes security and style. Both are associated with upscale items, such as jewelry, clothing, and appliances. These metallic colors are often used as accents.

Wear gold to exude warmth and silver to evoke strength of character.

As you explore the beautiful world of color, become purposeful in introducing the ones that impact you in the most positive way and to influence how you feel. Integrate the right colors into your daily life for maximum joy and harmony. When used effectively, color can really brighten up your day and your life. We have talked about the color black being the most slimming in the color spectrum. However, any color that looks good on you, when worn head to toe, will give a similar effect. The trick is to figure out which colors look best on you.

It can be utterly confusing.

Besides, there are so many shades of every color in the spectrum. There isn't just one shade of blue, red, yellow, or green. Blue can be navy blue, ice blue, bright blue, or a seafoam blue. Some of these are cold, and some are warmer.

You may not think that a certain color suits you, but there will always be a shade that will suit you, so open up your imagination and experiment. You may be pleasantly surprised.

FIND THE RIGHT SHADES THAT FLATTER

How to pick the colors that look best on you and which ones to kiss goodbye and banish from your wardrobe forever? Here is a simple process that will help you narrow down the colors that flatter you.

First go to your wardrobe and pull out the clothes in the colors you wear most often, the ones you tend to reach out to almost always. We're only looking at colors, not the fit of your clothes, so we can determine how the precise shades work with your face.

THE MIRROR EXERCISE

Separate piles of the different colors: reds in one pile, blues in another, greens in the third, and so on and so forth. Then take one pile at a time to a full-length mirror in good daylight. Hold each piece against your face and see what it does.

Does your skin glow or does it look sallow? Do your eyes look brighter or do your dark circles look worse? Does the color wash you out and match your hair color too much? Which shade looks best?

Once you have gone through all the piles and tested all the different colors in all the shades, you will have the final pile of the shades that suit you best.

Now go over the process once again. Let's say you have the blues, the greens, the reds, the yellows, etc. in the shades that look best on you; your next step is to determine which of these different *colors* look better on you.

DOMINANT VS. ACCENT COLORS

Now we will find your dominant colors. Dominant colors are colors that are most flattering on you. These will be the primary colors you will wear. For instance, green may look fine, but blue makes you look *so much more* attractive.

Take each color from the pile you had sorted out and stand in front of the mirror. Hold each color against your face. First one color, then another, and compare. You will go through every color and compare. It will be immediately apparent to you which colors are right for you.

Once you have established which color category you fall in, you might find that blues and reds flatter you the most, that they look better than the shades of greens or yellows that you had initially decided were flattering.

If that's the case, then blue and red are your dominant colors. And green and yellow are your accent colors. The accent colors will look great as an accessory or in a scarf or detail, or even as secondary colors to wear when you are feeling extra confident.

Now you are able to make wise choices. This will help you the next time you go shopping so that you don't make any impulse purchases. You want colors in your wardrobe that enhance your personality and flatter your skin tone.

Of course, blacks and whites are a must in every woman's wardrobe. These are two colors that are classic and suit everyone. Although, there are shades of white and shades of black that you may want to pay attention to as well.

White can be sharp and bright, or it can be creamy, like ecru. A shade of white may have a wonderfully uplifting effect on you, lighting up your eyes and giving a natural reflection to your face, while another shade will totally wash you out.

The same goes for black. It is said there are at least fifty shades of black, so make sure you choose wisely.

When in doubt, do *the mirror exercise* again and again, and you will know.

WARM VS. COOL COLORS

Understanding warm versus cool is pretty straightforward and intuitive. Warm colors are the stuff of fire and sunlight—red, yellow, and orange. Cool colors are blue, green, or violet.

Given common hair, eye, and skin color combinations, most people look best in shades from one side of the spectrum or the other.

The best way to type yourself is by testing out with metallics. Warm types look best in gold jewelry while cool types shimmer in silver. To test your color temperature, buy foil paper in gold and in silver and hold a piece of each below your face. Which one brings out the glow?

YOU'RE SUITED TO COOL COLORS

If your skin has more blue undertones and burns easily. In this case, along with blues and greens that look great on you, opt for black, gray, and deep gem tones. The best reds for you will be the blue-reds, such as eggplant or burgundy.

DO WEAR: Black, strong purples, darker shades of gray. Navy is good only when teamed up with turquoise or emerald greens. Icy-pale colors look good, too, as long as they are not teamed with black.

AVOID: Rust, dull apricot, beige, and any shade of brown.

YOU'RE SUITED TO WARM COLORS

If your hair and eyes could be described as "earthy." If warm colors give you that glow, then rich spice colors all work for you, as does gold jewelry. Pastels tend to make your skin look sallow or clash with your hair.

DO WEAR: Autumnal colors such as rusts, khakis, warm rich browns, olive greens, and tomato reds. Brick as long as it's not too pink. Blue as long as it's more of a teal blue.

AVOID: Black, navy, gray, pastel blue, any shade of pink.

Colors that are cold or have too much blue in them, such as hot pink or bright turquoise, are not recommended.

You could still be warm and not suit apricot. But if you don't suit olive and mustards then you don't belong in the warm category at all.

YOU'RE IN-BETWEEN AND MID-TONE:

Chances are your skin tone falls somewhere between the extremes of blue and yellow undertones, or you're neutral. In that case you have a lot of flexibility with color. When in doubt, it helps to judge a hue by how it brings out your eyes, not your skin.

DO WEAR: Purples, especially wisteria and lavender, soft blue, sage green, dark lavender, navy, periwinkle, burgundy, warm pastels like powder pink or blue.

AVOID: Stay away from all very cold bright colors such as blue-red, cardinal purple, and dull shades of beige and khakis.

Granted, green is always cooler than yellow. But you can find cooler or warmer tones within a color group that work best for you. For example, a cool pink is more lilac, and a warm pink is more on the peachy side. Red is cooler if it has more of the violet undertones and warmer if it's closer to orange.

If you get the color mix right, your wardrobe will be free of those annoying items that don't look good with anything else. You will no longer agonize over what to wear, and you will save money because you will shop smarter.

You will look more alive, your eyes will shine, and not only will *you* begin to see a difference but also people around you will start to comment on how well you look.

Don't be too conservative. Wear that strong color or that bold accessory and make your statement.

Don't be afraid to stand out. Be afraid not to.

"The best color in the whole world is the one that looks good on you."

—Coco Chanel

CHAPTER NINE

ORGANIZING YOUR CLOSET

You are certain you have a flared skirt and a cashmere T somewhere, if only you could find them. You've stood in front of your closet on too many mornings and felt the panic rising.

You know you've made some brilliant purchases, but they seem to have disappeared while sharing space with a riot of clutter and a league of has-beens. Added to these is a crew of wrong-sized items that you've been holding onto for when you will shed those extra pounds that crept up when you were not paying attention.

Somewhere between casual Fridays and suiting separates, between sleeveless dressing and bundling up because the temperature dropped while you were too busy with life to notice, things got a little confusing.

Now you feel like you have to go shopping because you have nothing to wear. All that chaos in your wardrobe is driving you insane! But you find shopping about as much fun as a root canal, and impulse buys are starting to drain your retirement fund.

Take a deep breath and shop your closet first before rushing out to make more purchases that will only be piled on top of what you already own.

The following four-step closet overhaul will make you a sort-and-purge enthusiast in no time at all. But before you start the process you may want to seek help. Don't do it alone. Make sure you have a friend to harden your resolve.

The friend you seek help from must be compulsively honest, and if she's not your size and shape, so much the better—or she will want your clothes and may have an ulterior motive when telling you something doesn't look great on you. Her honest opinion will be critical as you decide what looks good on you and what to discard, donate, resell, or give away.

Have on hand a full-length mirror, labels, lots of hangers, a bag of heavy-duty garbage bags, and a rolling rack if possible.

Now you're ready to edit your wardrobe, organize, and take control.

1. SEPARATE AND CREATE ORDER

Move your off-season clothes, shoes, scarves, etc. out or to the back of your closet. This is the stuff that you do not need this season. Don't just dump them, but store them correctly. Make sure they are clean, as insects such as moths are attracted to dirt and odors.

Make five piles:

- Clothes to be tossed.
- Items you want to keep.
- Items that need attention (such as to be cleaned or tailored).
- Pieces you will donate to charity.
- Items you want to resell.

2. STORE AND ORGANIZE

Here are some organizing tips and tricks to help you find what you need quickly.

Line your drawers with paper, or get plastic dividers. Old shoeboxes will do as well.

UNDERWEAR
Divide your bras and underwear by style and color: for everyday, evening, or sport.

SOCKS AND TIGHTS
Keep stockings separate from socks, dark colors from light, in categories of style and warmth. Throw away any that have runs or holes. Make sure they're all clean and ready for use.

SCARVES
Separate the ones you rarely use. Fold them and put them in baskets, placing the fragile scarves, those in silk and cashmere, in shallow drawers or in their own storage boxes with lids and labels. Scarves that you use consistently can be folded over a tie rack on the doors of the wardrobe or on wide hangers. You want to make sure they are visible so you can remember to wear them.

BELTS
These can be hung on a row of hooks at eye level to make them easy to reach, or even over the hooks of hangers with the outfits you normally wear them with.

JEWELRY
You can have a bulletin board on the back of your closet door and pin necklaces and earrings on it. Boxes are fine for bracelets and items you wear on special occasions only as long as they are kept sparse to avoid being tangled or crushed.

BAGS AND PURSES
Have these rest upright and lined up on a shelf or in cubbyholes by size and color. Those used for special occasions can be stored in their own bags and labeled. Stuff them with tissue paper to maintain their shape.

FOOTWEAR

The ideal solution is to place these on a shoe rack. Built-in shelves or hanging canvas shelves are also perfect. However, if you lack space then store them in clear boxes or in their original boxes with a photo of them taped to the front. Keep them polished and clean. Use shoe trees or stuff them with paper to hold the shape.

3. HANG AND FOLD

Hanging clothes in an orderly fashion is the secret to getting the most mileage out of your wardrobe.

First of all, toss out all those wire hangers and invest in coordinating, slim, preferably padded wooden or plastic hangers that are not slippery and that don't slope too much.

Subdivide outfits by color then by style and fabric. Group outfits in colors that go together, from light to dark. Skirts should be with skirts, pants with pants, dresses with dresses. If space is small you may want to consider double-hanging rods above and below for shirts and pants.

Fold neatly all your T-shirts, sweaters, and cardigans, and stack in gradations of color, on shelves and in piles that are not too high, leaving some space between each pile. Narrow piles allow for easy access, neatness, and good visibility.

Buy bins or baskets to hold swimsuits, sweats, and exercise gear.

Jeans do not need to be hung. They can be folded and stored neatly on shelves, as it matters little if they are crushed.

Scatter your shelves with fragrant cinnamon sticks, cloves, or lavender bags to help keep moths at bay. Moths love wool and cashmere and clothes that are food-encrusted, so make sure never to put away a garment that is dirty or soiled.

4. SCAN YOUR WARDROBE

You're close. Just follow this final step to enjoy your get-happy closet.

Now that you have sorted everything and organized your closet you can scan your wardrobe for any excess or shortages.

Do you need more basics and less thrills and frills?

Is your wardrobe filled with prints and not enough solids? Too many blacks and whites and not enough color?

Would having a few more blouses help increase your options with the pants and skirts you already own? Or is there a certain skirt you think would be great to have, considering all the beautiful shirts you could wear it with?

Perhaps more metallic colors and lacy camisoles are needed to round out your wardrobe?

Is there a need for more variety, seeing that your outfits are all too predictable and similar? Maybe a couple more silhouettes would be great to have to add to the mix?

Make a list of items you feel you need to make your wardrobe more interesting and complete. Get inspired with the options you have and create outfits by pairing different tops with different bottoms, shoes, and jewelry.

Just as designers do at runway shows and in their design studios, whereby they have look books and inspiration boards, you too could take pictures of your outfits and create your own look book. In this book you will have pictures of your ideal outfits in the combinations you love. You can revisit your photo collection again and again to see different ways of wearing your clothes, and how the various pieces you own can be paired. This book will inspire you and be used as a guide on days when you feel rushed, lost, and confused.

This is the final step in your organizing venture. As the fog clears, you will feel as if you have more clothes and do not need to splurge on items that are unnecessary. You will learn to differentiate your wants from your needs. And in the process, you will save a whole lot of money!

Not only that, but you will feel a sense of peace and well-being descend upon you. Know that your outer world impacts your inner world, and external clutter creates inner chaos that may subtly diminish and blatantly rob you of your sense of well-being. In doing your "spring cleaning" and organizing your closet, you are in essence not only working on yourself from the outside in but also from the inside out.

Best of all, you can now spend more time doing other things that are more important and be more productive in life.

Congratulations on a job well done!

THINGS I NEED TO GET RID OF:

_____

_____

_____

_____

_____

_____

_____

_____

_____

_____

_____

_____

_____

_____

_____

_____

_____

_____

_____

_____

ITEMS I NEED TO ADD TO MY WARDROBE:

_____
_____
_____
_____
_____
_____
_____
_____
_____
_____
_____
_____
_____
_____
_____
_____
_____
_____
_____
_____
_____
_____
_____
_____
_____

"Opening up your closet should
be like arriving at a party
where everyone you see
is someone you like"

—Amy Fine Collins

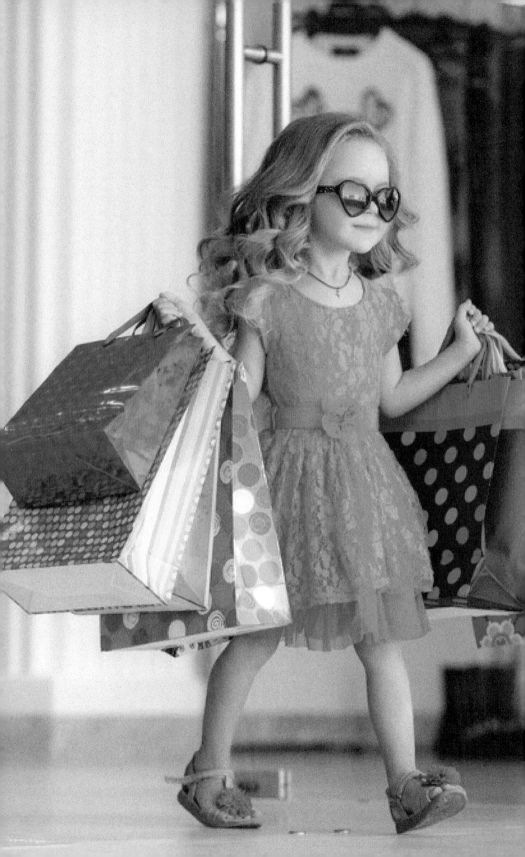

CHAPTER TEN

"Happiness is not in money but in shopping."
—*Marilyn Monroe*

Now that your closets are organized and your wardrobe edited to suit your needs, it's time to replenish and add items you feel are missing and which you feel would complement what you already own.

Add to that list a few items that you feel would enhance your lifestyle and personality.

To have your ultimate perfect wardrobe, you need a plan.

The List: Scan the list you made, determine exactly what you need, and only look for those items you have listed. Differentiate between your needs and your wants so you don't get too carried away.

Accessories: This is the magic wand that turns everything it touches into gold. Accessories complete your look; they add personality, color, and texture to your attire, allowing you to have a smaller wardrobe and yet be able to dress for any occasion. Most importantly, accessories help with your figure priorities. They tend to draw attention to areas you want to enhance, and at the same time take focus away from areas you're sensitive about. Having the right accessories in your closet means that you do not need to splurge on too many clothes.

Locations to shop: Study where, in your area, would be the best places to go to pick up the different items on your list. For instance, Neiman Marcus may boast to have the best lingerie experts in your area, and you know you could use their assistance and expertise, so that is where you would go for your lingerie. The shoes you are looking for in the price you can afford may be available at Nordstrom's, so that is where you would go for your shoes. Your pantsuits and dresses may be available at Saks Fifth Avenue and you know a salesperson there who has always been wonderful in helping you find the best at the most affordable prices, so off you go for those items to Saks. You get the drift . . .

Do Your Homework: Look at magazines to see what is being featured currently or ask friends and coworkers where they purchased items that you have admired. Make sure you're not getting carried away with overly trendy items, as they may be out of style even before you have a chance to show off yours. Have tear sheets and printouts of these items as reference and see how they fit in with your plan and your list.

Set a Budget: Set an overall budget and stick to it. Make up your mind that you will not go over, or if you feel compelled to because an item suits you so well, that it will not be more than 10 percent of your allocated dollars. Stop shopping once you hit the limit.

Look for Sales: Stores constantly slash prices, sometimes by up to 70 percent, to get rid of seasonal merchandise and to make room for new collections. However, competition can be fierce, and you must have a plan or you will lose out to more talented shoppers. To be sale-ready, follow these steps:

- *Make a list*: List the items you need that are on sale. If some of them are on sale online then the minute the sale starts make sure you are prepared to buy. If it's at the store then be there as soon as the sale starts or they'll run out of sizes and colors you're looking for. Only go to sales of designers or stores you love.

- *Always buy the right size*: Even before the sale starts go into the store to determine which size you will need, as each manufacturer has different fits and size charts. You may be a 4 in Calvin Klein but an 8 in Armani. Make sure of your size to avoid disappointment. Some sale items are final and nonrefundable, so do your homework. If you're buying online then know your bust, hips, and waist measurements so you can compare your size to their size charts.

- *Have the right foundation on*: Be prepared to make a decision by having the proper undergarment on so you know exactly how the garment will fit.

- *Get on mailing lists*: Sign up with stores you're interested in so that when items you covet go on sale you're one of the first to know. You can get advance notice and the inside scoop for when sales happen. By subscribing to their social media you could even get a twenty-four-hour head start before they open the sale to the public.

- *Act quickly*: If you've found what you want then act immediately. If you want choices then you'll need to be at the stores early to avoid losing out on your colors and sizes, and to avoid the long lines that are normal at sales. If you're shopping an online sale, rather than be beaten by other more savvy shoppers and see the big bargain disappear because someone beat you to the checkout, buy the item you want before going back to browse for more online.

- *Don't buy it just because it's on sale*: A red tag with "70 percent" written on it can work magic on your brain. Don't let yourself be carried away; instead, ask yourself: "Would I buy it if it weren't on sale? Do I actually love it?" If the answer is no, then walk away. It's not an investment piece if it just sits at the bottom of your wardrobe never to be worn.

Happy shopping!

"DON'T BUY IT JUST BECAUSE IT'S ON SALE"

—Rani St. Pucchi

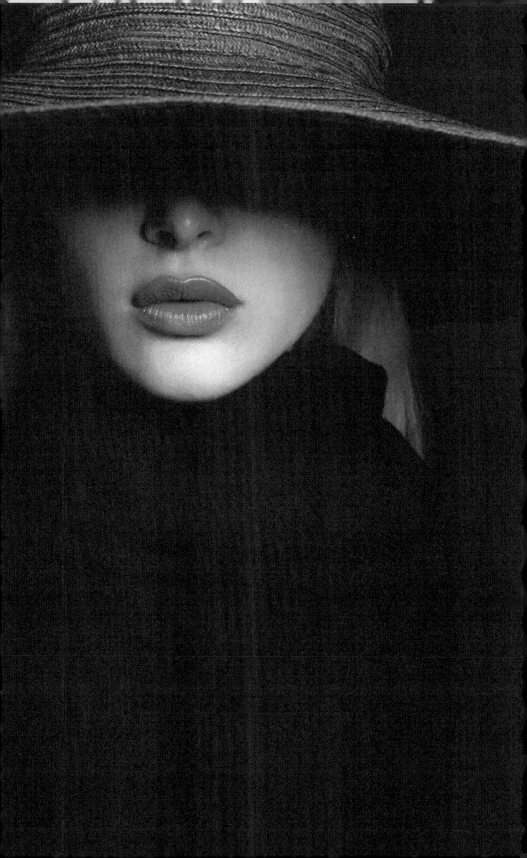

CHAPTER ELEVEN

DEFINING YOUR PERSONAL STYLE

"Be yourself. Everyone else is taken."
—Oscar Wilde

We live in a world that seduces us to be like everyone else. The influence and hypnosis we experience through the social media, fashion magazines, and society to buy certain things, to dress a certain way, and to conform so we can belong is overpowering.

Worse still is the advice given out by style books to change the way we dress after a certain age. Women over forty, and especially those over fifty, are told to wear more subdued clothing and dress more conservatively—that they should cover up their arms, lengthen their skirts, and avoid bold prints and exuberant colors.

Personally, I feel that the most important aspect about style is to do what suits *your* personality and meets your personal preferences. It really is *your* choice.

Being original, being authentic, being yourself, and standing in your own truth—that is true power. Therefore it is extremely important that you understand your own personal style.

Style is that hard-to-define word that describes how you

present yourself to the world. It is an expression of individualism mixed with charisma, an effortless confidence that you exude in being yourself, a magic wand that transforms you into a unique being.

Your style reflects who you are. It is very personal and unique to you. It is the way you dress that makes you happy, confident, and beautiful. In the process it matters not how many people you please as long as you are pleased with yourself. And it all starts with what you wear and how you present yourself to the world.

Does your wardrobe say something about you?

Chances are there's a style definition that resonates with you. You respond to certain styles better than others and some pieces just feel right when you put them on.

Look in your wardrobe and what do you see? At one end you see rows of clothes you wear every day because you love them all, but at another end are stacks and rows that you pass. If you're not wearing everything you've got then something is not right.

Does your wardrobe work together? If not, wouldn't now be the time to assess who you are, what your personality is, and what you wish to convey to the world? Are you happy with what you see? Does what you wear make you feel beautiful and give you effortless confidence? Knowing who you are and what you want to project through your personal style is what empowers you.

While it is true that some people are naturally very stylish and know how to combine clothes to create looks that are cohesive, effortless, and chic, most women are not born with this skill. But this does not mean that they cannot have lots of style.

As with anything, practice makes perfect. When you want to learn how to play the piano you will need to practice every single day to become very good at it. The same is true for wannabe authors; they must write every single day. Thus it is that style only gets better with age as we naturally learn daily what looks and feels good as we dress and style ourselves every single day.

It can work wonders to learn a few tricks and understand your body, balance, and how clothing and grooming can work to enhance your style. Feeling better about yourself and the way you look can change your life.

Create your own individual and visual style. Let it be unique for yourself and yet identifiable for others. After all, we live in a visual world. It's what people see first before they even know you well, that they form their opinions on. Unlike fashion, which changes constantly and fades over time, style is eternal. There is no separation between you as a woman, your clothes, and your way of being. Finding that unique style that works just for you can be magical indeed!

If you're struggling with finding your unique style start by following the few simple steps listed here until you feel confident and adventurous enough to venture outside your comfort zone:

- Find out what body type you have by measuring yourself and referring to the chart in Chapter One. Look for what suits your body type and what silhouettes you should avoid.

- Mix and experiment with patterns, keeping it simple at first by combining minimalist, high quality clothes in enduring colors.

- Have basics and essentials in your wardrobe that you can dress up or dress down. These are your basic camisoles, shirts, skirts, and pants.

- When mixing colors stick to trusted combinations such as black and white, navy and white, cream and caramel

- Wear dresses. Adding simple shift dresses in good fabrics to your wardrobe means you only need to worry about one garment and there is no need to mix and match. Dress it up with simple jewelry or a belt that will always make you look stylish.

- Add accessories to your wardrobe. Your clothes can be easily transformed with the right accessories. Keep them simple and minimalistic at first.

- Pay attention to grooming. Having well-manicured nails and a good haircut always elevates your style.

- Wear clothes that fit your personality, ones that

suit you and make you feel more confident.

- Start adding your *signature* to every outfit. This could be the way you wear your scarf, a hat, belt, or jewelry.

Pay attention to what fashion you are drawn to by observing people around you, or referring to ads in fashion magazines. This will allow you to experiment more and find out what works for you and what doesn't. Keep a scrapbook or pin the styles that inspire you. Whenever you see others wearing clothes you like and admire try to get a picture and paste it on your Pinterest board.

What comfort level is important to you? Which cut and silhouette appeals to you? Do you like timeless or trendy, prints or solids? After a while, you will see a pattern developing of the kind of styles that you like.

Over time you will realize that you have acquired a way of dressing that resonates with your personality, that you feel good in, and that boosts your self-confidence. Once you've identified the components of your style, only follow the latest trends that fit your style, and develop it until you have mastered your unique look.

You will now realize that you are making fewer buying mistakes, that you feel more at ease around people and your environment, that you are able to communicate with more confidence, and that you start to give a clear message to others about who you are through your clothes and your personal style.

So, perhaps vintage Valentino and Chanel haute couture are not your personal favorites, and you prefer a more casual look.

Here's a lineup of style categories that may resonate best with your personality.

GIRL NEXT DOOR

You like sporty-chic and youthful basics. Minimalism and simplicity are your signature style. You're all about owning less and enjoying the things you have more. That is why it's more important for you to buy the right clothes, clothes that are of better quality and that fit you extremely well. You prefer the fresh, young, yet proper look, and you could care less for the show-everything-and-layer-it-on trend. For special occasions, you love feminine, fitted dresses, but you keep jewelry to a bare minimum.

The message you give others is that you are easygoing and that you like a simple and carefree way of life.

NATURAL, ALL-AMERICAN

You love fashion, but you choose clothes that exude comfort. Whether you're wearing a simple tank and skirt, or a vintage Chanel, you look cool without being contrived. There's no excess, no confusion, and the focus is always on your natural assets. On those special occasions and evenings out, you're just as comfortable and confident with those plunging Vs and statement jewelry worn in a sleek, uncluttered way. Your way of dressing is classic, timeless, and enduring.

You let others know that you are the fun-without-the-fuss kind of gal. You like the finer things in life as long as they are not complicated and dramatic.

BOHEMIAN

You are an expert at spinning a look with a vintage extra or a slightly unexpected and out-of-the-norm pairing. You have a nonconforming style that tends to be associated with the hippie era. There's a little gypsy in your soul that shows itself in how masterfully you accessorize and mix pieces. You like making sound with your chunky jewelry and revel in the statement you make with your big, unstructured bags, your boots, and your vintage jeans and jackets.

You exude a carefree, timeless, and organic spirit filled with creativity and celebration. You are playful and thrive in nature, rest, and relaxation.

GLAMOROUS

More is more, and too much is never enough. You have a no-holds-barred look, but this look doesn't happen by accident. There's careful planning and a method to your style. You tend to be trendy, fashionable, and willing to take risks, and you are happy to stand out. You flourish in your femininity, not just by keeping your look electric but by making sure your clothes and colors flatter your body. You have style and know well how to combine jeans and mink together and rock them like no other woman could.

You come across as a woman of culture, fashion, and sensuality.

LADYLIKE

You have a polished and a very "done" look that is elegant yet personal. You know how to elevate an elegant suit by adding a creative personal signature, like a shot of color in your shoes, a single standout piece of jewelry, or an antique hairpin. You have a good eye for what you like, know what suits you, and have the innate instinct or (learned) knowledge to mix it all together. You have a very creative and fun way of dressing. You exude confidence in your every action, in how you walk, how you talk, and how you dress.

Others see you as a well-learned, polished woman, exuding wealth and comfort with genuine elegance.

If you are like most women, you will have elements of a few of these styles within your own personal and unique style. You may gravitate towards classic garments and go for a minimal look, yet love fashion, new trends, and new colors. Bohemian style may not be your "thing," but occasionally you find yourself wearing chunky jewelry and vintage attire.

Once you have discovered your unique personal style, you can start to refine it by applying some general principles of silhouette, playing with colors and textures and discovering the ones that suit you best. Finding your own unique style and advancing it to the next level is an exciting journey of discovery.

Knowing your personal style helps remove the guesswork in how you shop and what you ultimately allow to hang in your closet. There is no risk of impulse purchases as you run through your style filter to hone in only on those items that say something about you. There is no more confusion as you allow your personality to shine. You can then step out in style in the certain knowledge that you look and feel great, and most of all you're having fun in the process!

"Fashion is an expression of faith. In this world of ours that seeks to give away its secrets one by one, that feeds on false confidences and fabricated revelations, it is the very incarnation of mystery, and the best proof of the spell it casts is that, now more than ever, it is the topic on everyone's lips."

—*Christian Dior, 1956*

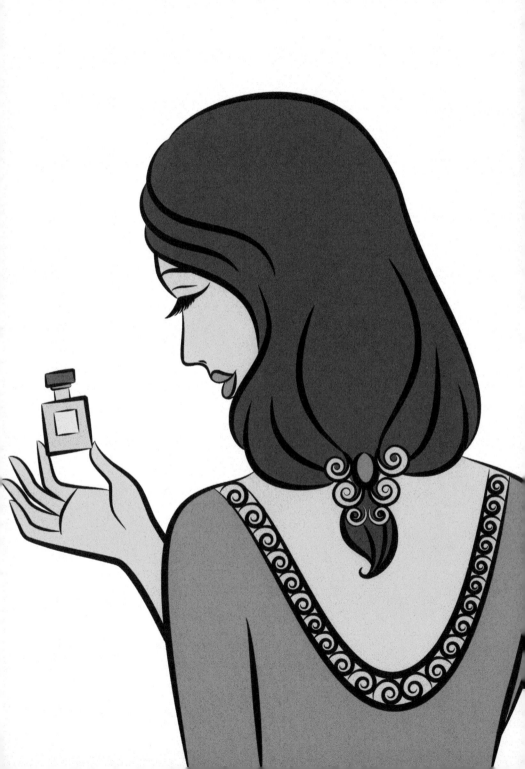

CHAPTER TWELVE

SCENT OF A WOMAN

Scent of a Woman is a 1992 American drama film produced and directed by Martin Brest. I just loved the movie and thought the title seemed appropriate for what I am addressing in this chapter.

There seem to be so many conflicting theories about perfumes that I felt a whole chapter needed to be dedicated to this subject.

Other than your style, the scent you wear speaks volumes about you and your personality. Smells are about pure pleasure, as they speak differently to our emotional brains. They evoke memories and buried emotions, often transporting us to times that were happy or sad. Knowing this, it helps to find a scent that takes you to your happy place, filled with love and joy.

Be cautious about purchasing perfume just because it smells good on someone else. Each body translates the same scent differently. Try the scent before you buy by wearing it for at least a couple of hours, or even a whole day, so you'll know how it unfolds and whether you still love it.

DIFFERENT TYPES OF PERFUMES:

Shopping for new perfume can be overwhelming. Not only are there countless scents available; there are also different fragrance concentrations. Underneath the name of the perfume on a bottle will normally be the fragrance concentration.

A fragrance concentration refers to the strength that a fragrance has. Perfumes with a higher fragrance concentration contain more perfume oils and less alcohol.

You will typically see five different kinds of perfumes: parfum, eau de parfum, eau de toilette, eau de cologne, eau fraiche.

Fragrance concentrations are broken into the following main categories:

Parfum:
This is the most concentrated and pure form of perfume. It contains anywhere from 15 percent to 40 percent fragrance; however, the concentration is generally between 20 to 30 percent. Of all scents, parfums last the longest, usually six to eight hours. Parfum generally also commands the highest price of all the fragrance types due to the high concentration of fragrance. People with sensitive skin may do better with parfums as they have far less alcohol than other fragrance types and therefore are not as likely to dry out the skin.

Eau de Parfum:
After parfum, eau de parfum has the next highest concentration of fragrance. It typically contains up to 20 percent perfume oil. On average, eau de parfum will last for four to five hours. It's also generally less expensive than parfum, and while it does have a higher concentration of alcohol than parfum, it is better for sensitive skin than other fragrance types. Eau de parfum is one of the most common fragrance types and is suitable for everyday wear.

Eau de Toilette:
The term eau de toilette came from the French term "faire sa toilette" which means getting ready. Eau de toilette is the lightest-

wearing scent with only about 5 percent to 15 percent of the essential fragrance. It is cheaper than eau de parfum and is one of the most popular types of fragrances available. EDT fragrance will normally last for two to three hours. Eau de toilette is ideal for daywear while eau de parfum is best for nightwear.

Eau de Cologne:

Eau de cologne has a much lower concentration of fragrance than the above types of perfume. It generally has a 2 to 4 percent concentration of fragrance and a high concentration of alcohol. It is less expensive than other types of fragrance; however, the scent generally only lasts for up to two hours. Eau de cologne generally comes in bigger bottles, as more of the fragrance needs to be used.

Eau Fraiche:

Eau fraiche is similar to eau de cologne in that the scent will generally last for up to two hours. It has an even lower concentration of fragrance than eau de cologne, normally only 1 to 3 percent. While eau fraiche has a low fragrance concentration, it does not contain a high amount of alcohol. Along with the fragrance, the remainder of eau fraiche is mostly water.

Along with the types of perfume listed above, there are mists, aftershaves, and other types of fragrances available. Higher-end fragrances can cost a significant amount of money, so doing research beforehand will ensure that you get the type of fragrance you are looking for.

HOW TO APPLY PERFUME SO IT LASTS:

> "'Where should one use perfume?' a young woman asked. 'Wherever one wants to be kissed,' I said."
> —Coco Chanel

So how do you apply perfume to make it last all day? This is a question often asked by most women. It turns out that there are areas on the body that are best for spritzing—and they are not always the places we expect.

The most optimum body areas are pulse points, including wrists and backs of the knees, as well as areas such as the belly button, which emit heat and maximize scent intensity.

Hair

Fragrances latch onto fibers, which is why the strands of your hair will carry the scent of perfume for a long-lasting effect. Hair fibers are optimum for clutching onto the perfume's particles. The fragrance will also cling onto any products you've used after washing your hair, perfect for a subtle finish.

The alcohol content present in perfume can dry out the hair, so rather that spritzing directly onto strands, mist onto a brush or comb and delicately pull through.

Ears

Spray your scent of choice behind the ear lobes: this area is a pulse point, where the body is warmer, which will serve to enhance the fragrance.

Additionally, for an amplified effect, try the area at the tops of your ears, as skin tends not to dry out there.

Collarbone & Décolletage

Maximize the power of your perfume by giving your collarbone and décolletage (neck, shoulders, and back) a spritz.

The dips in the bone structure will see perfume more likely to settle there, and the added bonus of wearing strappy tops and plunging necklines means there's extra surface area to exude fragrance from.

Wrists

Hands carry pulse points that emit fragrance strongly. Apply fragrance on the wrists, as they serve as a pulse point and area of enhanced heat to further amplify the scent. For those who are expressive talkers, give the backs of hands a gentle dab with the fragrance, to get your perfume noticed in transit.

Inside Elbows
Another pulse point is the inside of the elbows, which as well as emitting the enhanced fragrance, serves to slightly obscure the smell in the bends of the arms—perfect for longer-lasting diffusion. Maximize the power of the perfume by ensuring skin is moisturized, as the more hydrated your skin is, the longer the fragrance will last.

Behind Knees
As well as being another area where veins rise close to the skin, the backs of the knees are warmer and softer, and therefore more likely to project the scent.
The area behind the knees is perfect to carry fragrance for a long-lasting effect, and perfect for summer, emitting your fragrance of choice with every crossing and uncrossing of legs.

Feet
An area of the body that is in perpetual motion, spraying calves and spritzing on ankles with perfume is not only refreshing, but will help to waft your fragrance wherever you go.

Belly Button
The belly button is a surprising area of the body that holds fragrance well, due to its warmth. Practically a receptacle for scent, this is a must if you're baring your midriff or sporting a bikini. Put little drops on your fingers and apply in your belly button. When you apply fragrance to areas where you heat up, the smell stays with you.

Clothing
For additional perfume power, summer wraps and pashminas will retain fragrances beautifully, as the scent particles clutch onto the fibers.

FINDING THE RIGHT FRAGRANCE

Choosing the right perfume for you and your personality can be tough. If you've never worn perfume before or you're just in the market for a new fragrance, the choices can overwhelm you. Do you go fruity and floral or opt for something muskier? Deciding on a signature scent comes down to personal preference and can take time.

Determining the very best fragrance for you, one that tells the world who you are, takes some finesse and a full engagement of your senses. Before you choose a fragrance you need to know the basics as perfumes fall under several categories of scent.

What do you feel most called to?

Floral:
Perhaps the most popular scent option among women, floral perfumes contain the scent of either one flower (rose, gardenia, lavender) or a bouquet of several varieties. Floral scents are feminine and romantic.

Oriental:
These scents tend to be muskier and smell rich and slightly spicy with hints of vanilla, cinnamon, and clove.

Chypre:
These fragrances are warm and dry and almost all built around a woody, mossy accord of bergamot with hints of oak, moss, patchouli, and citrus. This family of perfumes is characterized by an earthy, woodsy scent.

Green:
This is an ideal light fragrance to be worn outdoors. Think fresh cut grass, crushed leaves, and other fresh, cool scents that bring to mind the outdoors and open spaces.

Fougère:
Fougère, which in French means fern, refers generally to fragrances that have a green accord through notes of lavender, sage, rosemary or other green-floral herbs, with a base like sandalwood or moss/musk to add depth. This family of scents is stronger and often used in men's fragrances.

Oceanic:
Popular among men, these scents are influenced by the sea and evoke being by the ocean (sandy beach, salty air). Oceanic scents are clean, almost masculine, with hints of spice and citrus.

Wood:
Exactly what it says. Feels like you have just stepped into a forest, as these are the notes you will get with a woody scent. Think cedar, pine, sandalwood—scents that are earthy and musky.

Are you confused yet?

Along with fragrance types there are also fragrance notes, which determine the final scent. With all of the types and scents available, shopping for perfume is not always easy, but it is possible given a little time and patience. And expert help is always available at perfume counters in high-end stores such as Barneys and Neiman Marcus, among others.

Your perfume should be as subtle as possible. When wearing perfume, make sure you don't go overboard. Less is more— especially when it's hot, as heat can intensify perfume on the skin and make it stronger than you intended.

"A woman's perfume tells more about her than her handwriting."

—Christian Dior

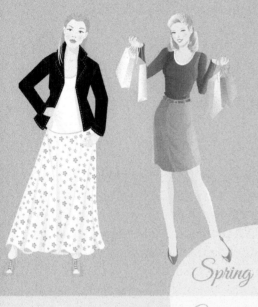
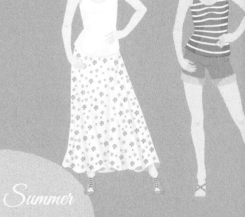
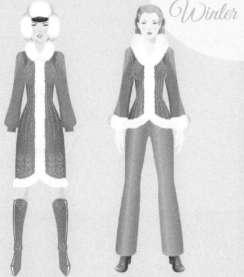
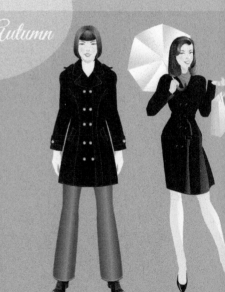

Spring   Summer

Winter   Autumn

CHAPTER THIRTEEN

WARDROBE FOR ALL SEASONS

"Baby, It's Cold Outside"
—a song written by Frank Loesser in 1944

When it comes to seasonal fashion most women suffer from angst and confusion called the seasonal affective disorder. What to wear, and when? With the global climate changing the way we dress, what used to be winter has turned into an unpredictable autumn, and spring sometimes never arrives, as we jump right into an eternal summer.

How to boost spring/summer basics to be as versatile and enduring as your fall/winter staples, and how to build a wardrobe to contain outfits you love, head to toe, can be a science.

Here are some suggestions, so lighten up!

SPRING/SUMMER:

Summer can be a challenging season to dress for many women. You reveal more of your body than in any other season and have fewer layering tricks at your disposal to cover up certain parts that you're not as comfortable with. Your wardrobe for this time of the year needs to be pretty flexible and hardworking.

Aside from needing to look appropriate as well as smart while remaining cool for work, there are PTA meetings or weddings to attend. The possibility of sudden changes in weather as well as last-minute beach weekends calls for fun and fundamental mix-and-match pieces, colors and prints, and spontaneity.

Have a wear-anywhere sundress? A camisole, a white T-shirt, or a cotton skirt you love? Now is the time to bring them out and enjoy them.

Here is a capsule wardrobe containing some versatile mix-and-match pieces to get you through this time of the year:

- Sundresses (a summer day dress and a high-summer beach dress)
- A work dress
- Evening black chiffon dress
- White T-shirt
- A classic men's white shirt: chic and simple
- Silk blouse
- Halter top
- Tank tops: cotton for day and dressy for evening
- Cotton shorts
- Camisole
- Khaki pants
- Flat-front lightweight mix cotton pants
- Cotton skirt
- A bias-cut or flowing skirt in chiffon
- Cotton cardigan or sweater
- Lightweight jacket or coat to cover up for rain or an evening chill
- Swimsuit

- Beach cover-up
- Thong sandals
- Open-toe work shoes and classic high-heel pumps
- Espadrilles
- Ballet flats
- Sunglasses
- Canvas tote
- Straw bag
- Evening clutch

You can dress these pieces up or down any which way you like. Add jewelry and accessories for an evening look to get out of being a bit too reliant on the humdrum shorts and a tired T. And for work, mix up those essential shapes and styles with a pair of open-toed heels, and you're ready to roll!

FALL/WINTER:

Tweed blazer? Check. Wool scarf? Check. Tall boots? Check. It's so easy to look smart at this time of the year. How wonderful it feels when ideas and plans come together in such harmony. When a wool coat looks just right with those boot-cut pants, or when the splurge-worthy shoes elevate a plum pencil skirt.

Here are some basics and ideas that can be combined into fresh and fabulous, smart outfits that can take you from a corporate meeting to an evening soirée effortlessly:

- Classic knee-length winter coat
- Casual all-weather jacket or a trench coat
- Wool blazer
- Non-seasonal wool pantsuit
- A-line or kick-pleat skirt
- Pencil or straight skirt

- Boot-cut black pants
- Flat-front wool trousers
- Chinos or cords
- Jacket to match skirt and pants
- Work dress
- Jersey wrap dress
- Little black dress
- Jeans: one dressy and one casual
- Turtleneck, V-neck, crew, and cardigan sweater
- White and black shirts
- Lightweight, chiffon, or silk blouse for evening (layer it!)
- Knee boots and ankle boots
- Ballet flats
- Black pumps and kitten heels
- Roomy work tote or hobo
- Structured handbag
- Evening clutch

Add to these your jewelry, accessories, scarves, and gloves, and you're ready to welcome fall and winter seamlessly and with confidence.

No matter what season you're dressing for, you can't skimp on the fundamentals if you're trying to build a perfect wardrobe. These are the essential underpinnings that can take you from season to season and from day into evening. Therefore, you'll want to buy basics in the best quality you can afford so you may have an ideal wardrobe for all seasons.

"I like my money
where I can
see it: hanging
in my closet."

—*Carrie Bradshaw*

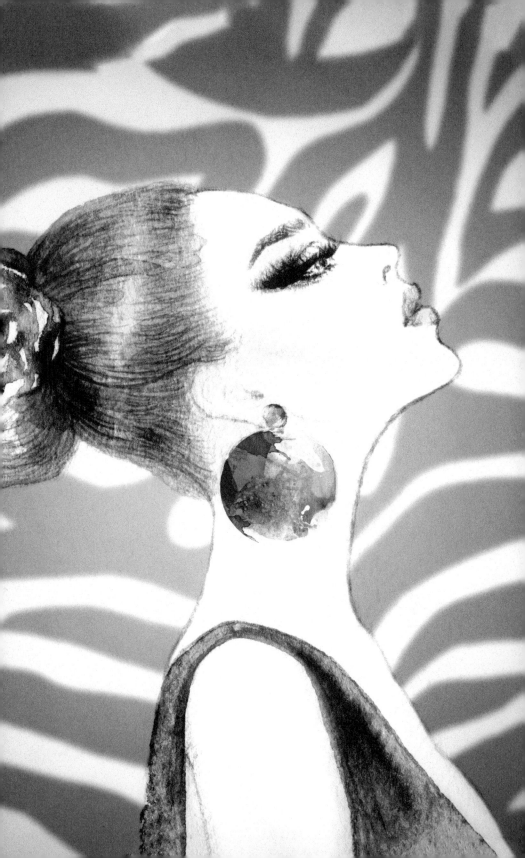

CHAPTER FOURTEEN

These 101 Styling Tips will further help you find, define, and elevate your style choices.

1. **Shirts with wide straps,** dresses and tops with higher necklines, three-quarter length sleeves are all very flattering on broad shoulders.

2. **To bring focus onto your waist** wear a belt that contrasts with your outfit. A dress or a top that wraps around or ties at your waist will draw the eye to your waist.

3. **To bring focus onto your bust** wear scoop or V-necklines, knits or soft fabrics, logistically placed prints or embellishment. A close-fit top, a peek-a-boo lace camisole, a slightly transparent top will all do the work.

4. **Styles that are slenderizing**: long vertical lines and patterns, tops with button-front closings, vertical tucks, and V-necklines. Skirts with vertical pressed pleats are also very slimming.

5. **Balance the plus or minus of your silhouette**. If your torso is narrow and your bottom broader, choose styles with details that broaden your top and vice versa.

6. **To minimize and downplay large areas** choose styles with virtually no details in the area you want to minimize. Also use dark solid colors in those larger areas and avoid large or horizontal prints and ruffles.

7. **Highlight areas you wish to flaunt** by choosing details such as draping, embellishments, pleats, and yokes that help accentuate those areas.

8. **To conceal certain areas** choose styles with a relaxed fit, and fabrics that flow. Avoid styles that are form-fitting and snug.

9. **To lift your mood** wear your favorite color.

10. **To look sexy** don clothes that bring focus on your strengths—tiny waist, cleavage, curved hips, elegant legs, or a combination of all if you're lucky.

11. **Don't keep repeating the same outfit** just because it's easy. Variety is the spice of life, so get out of the rut and experiment with different styles every now and then.

12. **To create an original look** take advantage of any family jewelry or an antique brooch you may have access to.

13. **If you're wearing dark colors** because you're feeling overweight and bloated, but the weather is hot, then make sure the fabric is lightweight.

14. **Camouflage a wide waist** with clothing that has no defined waistline, like a sheath dress or a tunic.

15. **For an instant artsy look**, wear a mid-calf skirt.

16. **A long heavy chain draped on a plunging neckline** will add weight to help hold the material in place while adding pizzazz.

17. **If you have heavy upper arms** you can still wear short sleeves as long as the sleeves are long enough to hide the heaviest part.

18. **The right hat can be your signature** and can help you look great on those bad hair days.

19. **Your sunglasses can make you feel chic instantly**. Pick out frames that suit your face.

20. **Wearing color** is the quickest way to get a compliment from a man.

21. **Your hem should never end at the thickest part of your leg**—be it above the knee, calf, or ankle. Adjust the hem to fall at a more slender part of your leg.

22. **Mix practicality with some femininity**. Wear a swinging georgette skirt with your suit jacket, or a lace camisole under your jacket.

23. **Have that one staple dinner dress** in which you feel great, so you never have to shop frantically to meet a last-minute invitation.

24. **When wearing a bold, bright color or print**, keep the line of the outfit simple to balance the drama.

25. **Sexy dressing might mean** wearing low-cut, short, or fitted clothes or baring shoulders, but unless you're comfortable it does not come across as attractive.

26. **Invest in the best handbag you can afford**. It will lift the level of your entire outfit with its message of quality and help your image.

27. **Your underwear should match your skin tone**, not the color of the clothes you wear.

28. **The prints you wear can reveal your personality**. A geometric print appears to be more orderly and predictable, while a wild print sends a message of excitement and flair.

29. **Soft textures** like chiffon, cashmere, and angora can feminize your outfit.

30. **Soft and thin fabrics** like silk crepe and wool jersey fall better and are more slenderizing than heavier and bulky fabrics like wool and tweed.

31. **When combining two different colors to wear**, choose the color that is more flattering of the two to wear next to your face.

32. **Wear high heels**, but never so high that you can't walk gracefully.

33. **If you have a tummy**, never wear a dress or a skirt that is too tight. A wrap skirt or one with a sarong tie is better.

34. **Purchasing a fragile item** means you must be willing to put up with the necessary upkeep, such as large cleaning bills and frequent ironing. Make your purchase decisions wisely.

35. **Make sure to match the colors of your outfits in daylight**. Different fabrics pick up the same dye shade differently.

36. **If you are short**, do not wear contrasting colors in one outfit but keep colors in one family instead. Contrasts break up height and make you look even shorter.

37. **If you are large**, avoid bold, expansive patterns and tiny floral prints. Also avoid fabrics that are too stiff or too flimsy.

38. **Before putting clothes back in your closet**, air them and make all necessary alterations so that every item is in tip-top shape and ready for wear when needed.

39. **Lacy lingerie** can slip you into a feminine mood and make you feel more confident.

40. **Except for your sweat suit**, be mindful that only your top or your bottom is loose and baggy, never both together.

41. **A wardrobe that consists of clothes in classic neutrals,** such as white, beige, gray, and black, will mix with anything. These can always be dressed up with colorful accessories, such as jewelry, belts, scarves, and jackets.

42. **When you are faced with a last-minute** date, dinner, or any special event and you have no time to change, a piece of jewelry and bright lipstick works beautifully. Keep these in your purse at all times.

43. **When shopping for new clothes or shoes** bear in mind that comfort should always come before fashion. If you have to keep pulling and adjusting no one will notice how good you look.

44. **When looking to exude authority**, closed pumps are more appropriate than open-toed shoes.

45. **Look for evening wear possibilities** in the lingerie department, such as a satin camisole or a lacy top. You can save a lot of money.

46. **A large colorful printed scarf** can serve as a hip wrap or a shawl as well as a brightener under your coat.

47. **A big white shirt** can be used as a cover-up for your bathing suit when tied at the waist or hip.

48. **If you feel your clothes are "running away" from your body** add a belt to secure the dress to your body.

49. **Have at least four to six favorite scarves** in different sizes and lengths, colors, and patterns in your wardrobe so you can change the mood of your outfits.

50. **When going on a trip**, pack basics for layering and unique pieces of jewelry to spice up your wardrobe to keep it interesting.

51. **If a certain designer's clothes fit you best** then stick to the designer and always check out their new collections. Designers tend to cut the same sizes and proportions over and over and even stick to similar fabrics in similar shades, making it easier to update your wardrobe.

52. **Dress weather-appropriate.** If it's raining, wear an outfit that goes with your "rainproof" shoes. If it's a cloudy day, wear a bright dress. If it's sunny and warm, wear your short flirty skirt or your light and softly draped dress. If it's hot, avoid your close-fitting suit.

53. **If a blouse or jacket** pulls around your shoulders and back even slightly, or if you can't button it, do not purchase it.

54. **Before going shopping** make a list of what you absolutely need and go straight for those items before spending all your money on other things.

55. **A bright accessory or a pair of shoes** with the latest shape or heel will update your entire wardrobe.

56. **Update your outfits** and give them a lift easily by shortening the hemline or changing the buttons on your shirt.

57. **Your jacket is the most important garment in your wardrobe.** Buy the best you can afford and make it a classic so it looks current for years to come.

58. **Invest in outfits that serve more than one function** and that can be dressed up or dressed down.

59. **Each new season buy one piece of clothing** that makes you feel current and that can mix easily with your existing wardrobe.

60. **Purchasing an inexpensive shirt or jacket** and changing to better quality buttons can transform it to look more expensive instantly.

61. **Your closet should be organized** so that every item is visible and uncovered to allow you to find what you need easily and instantly.

62. **In preparation for the next season** set aside time to clean out your closet and pack away what you will not need for the season. Fashion is synonymous with change. Keep only what you believe will be classic enough to look current the next season.

63. **The styles you love today may be outdated six months** from now, so don't collect too many articles in a similar style unless that is your signature.

64. **Don't save your clothes for that special occasion.** Enjoy all of them, as fashion can change, just as your body can change, over time.

65. **Don't ever** purchase clothes that you need help getting into.

66. **When shopping for specific clothing** bring along the right shoe, bra, or pieces you intend to wear with that item.

67. **Wear layers under a coat** to make sure it fits before purchasing it.

68. **When switching from day into evening**, wear your suit without a blouse.

69. **Have a couple of outfits in your favorite colors** that are your perk-me-ups to pull out and wear on days when you may be feeling sad or depressed.

70. **Remove the inside pocket lining** in pants and skirts to keep your clothes from bulging in the hips.

71. **Always have a black jacket and a black belt** in your wardrobe for an instantly pulled-together look.

72. **Looking authoritative** doesn't mean wearing drab and dull colors. Choose neutrals that are not mousy, not subtle, and not boring. Mix textures and add accessories to create style.

73. **When buying clothes and accessories**, keep in mind that any bra, skirt, or sleeve that is too tight and uncomfortable will keep you from being able to concentrate on your work or from looking confident.

74. **If you're wearing a matching color pant or skirt with the same color jacket**, your inside blouse or sweater should be a contrasting color.

75. **Do not wear dark underwear beneath light color outfits**. Even if you don't think you can see the contrast, others may be able to.

76. **To save yourself the trouble of checking your coat at restaurants and venues**, you may want to drape an evening shawl over your clothes instead. That way, you can keep it with you, and it can actually add a flash of color to your outfit as well.

77. **Cuffed pants** make your legs look shorter.

78. **Tucking your top into your pantyhose** helps give a smooth line and ensures it does not keep spilling out. You can still pull out your top evenly for that relaxed, blouson look.

79. **Make sure to stand up straight and tall**. Poor posture can ruin the look of your clothing.

80. **Too many grays and blacks in your wardrobe** give a sophisticated but drab message. Always introduce an interesting element or color to break it up.

81. **For effective storage**, take care to stuff your fragile blouse sleeves and evening gown sleeves with tissue paper. Stuff your strapped shoes, hats and pouch purses, as well, to maintain the shape.

82. **If you have a habit of slouching**, wear slightly higher heels to remind yourself to walk more gracefully.

83. **If you have a great rear**, wear bias-cut skirts in soft, flowy fabrics and well-fitted pants with tucked in tops.

84. **A pushed-up or rolled-up sleeve look** adds a modern twist to your jacket.

85. **Don't overdo it with the accessories**. They should never be the focus but lead the eye to your face instead.

86. **When at work**, avoid low necklines, clinging or see-through clothes, glitter, and tight-fitting outfits.

87. **Stay away from clinging fabrics if you are too thin**. Wear fabrics with some body instead.

88. **In the office or in your car**, always keep a pair of black pumps with the highest heels you feel comfortable walking in for unexpected dates or evenings out.

89. **If you admire a person for the way they look and dress**, it's perfectly okay to copy them. It could be their lipstick color, the way they layer their clothes, their impeccable way of dressing. The right role model is preferable to fashion magazines, which are all Photoshopped anyhow.

90. **Money spent on alterations is money well spent**. It saves you from having to purchase new expensive items of clothing each season and ensures that your outfits fit properly.

91. **Browsing through fashion in the best stores**, especially when your budget is small, means you can learn to look for similar merchandise at a more affordable store.

92. **When shopping, don't think you will lose weight and settle for a smaller size**. If it doesn't fit you now wait until you have lost the weight to make the purchase.

93. **Better to spend money on that one expensive item** rather than wasting money on a dozen compromises that do not give you as much joy.

94. **Your silk scarf can be your best friend**. Carry it in your bag to serve as a quick fix to dress up or add warmth to your outfit or as a cover for bare shoulders and neckline when needed.

95. **For a more balanced look**, wear the darker color on the bottom and keep the top lighter.

96. **When planning an outfit for an important occasion,** rehearse the entire outfit you're going to wear, exactly as you would wear it. Move around and sit down in it to make sure you will be comfortable. This will give you the confidence you need.

97. **Choose the outfit you're going to wear the night before.** This will help you make better decisions and ensure you don't freeze up in front of your closet in the mornings.

98. **Never make a purchase unless** the item says something you want to say about yourself.

99. **Comfort is key,** especially when you know you are going to a stressful event or will be having a long day. Make sure to choose the outfit and shoes that will keep you looking and feeling comfortable.

100. **Small, sophisticated geometric prints** give you a more authoritative look than do large prints and florals.

101. **Whatever you do, make sure your clothes fit** you well and look like they belong to you.

ABOUT THE AUTHOR

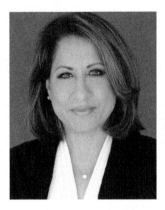

T hirty years ago, Rani St. Pucchi took the bridal world by storm, despite having no formal training in fashion. She is an award-winning couture fashion designer and founder of the world-renowned bridal house **St. Pucchi**. A passionate and dynamic entrepreneur who launched her global empire in the United States in 1985, Rani's vision was to create an avant-garde bridal and evening couture line modern in styling but classic in detail. That vision has been realized today.

Renowned for infusing her creations with touches of magnificently colored jewels, exquisite hand embroidery, delicate beading, and sparkling crystals on the finest silks and laces, these inspired designs with innovative draping evoke the timeless elegance every woman desires. As one of the foremost designers to introduce exotic silk fabrics and hand embroidery, Rani is applauded for being a pioneer in bringing color to the United States bridal scene, having learned that white does not flatter everyone.

Rani has been recognized and nominated on multiple occasions for her design talent and won numerous awards as Style Innovator. In addition, she has been honored with the Best Bridal Designer Award at the prestigious Chicago Apparel Center's Distinctive Excellence in Bridal Industry (DEBI) Awards.

Rani is famous for designing the wedding dress worn by Phoebe (Lisa Kudrow) as she captured the hearts of millions when she said "I do" in a unique *St. Pucchi* lilac corset bodice A-line gown on the finale of the hit television show **Friends**.

Her range of avant-garde designs are worn by the world's most discerning brides, including celebrities and style icons such as New York Giants' player Aaron Ross' wife, Olympic gold medalist, Sanya Richards; Dallas Cowboys' quarterback Tony Romo's wife, Candice Crawford; actress Tara Reid; Jason Priestley's wife, Naomi Lowde; actress Candice Cameron; and Grammy Award-winning country-music singer Alison Krauss, who donned a specially designed Chantilly lace and silk gown at the Country Music Awards.

Having distinguished herself in the upper echelons of luxury couture fashion, Rani has enjoyed much media attention. Her signature designs have been recognized in high-profile media spotlights such as *Entertainment Tonight, Harper's Bazaar, WWD, Town and Country, Bride's, Cosmopolitan Brides, Inside Weddings, Martha Stewart Weddings and The Knot.*

Rani's real passion other than the world of design is to help women who have suffered abuse, and who are struggling to find themselves. On her quest to empower women to be their best selves she is passionate about helping them find their voice through building their self-confidence. And as she rightfully notes, self-confidence must start with a woman's love and acceptance of her body.

Renowned for her savvy knowledge of a woman's form and fit, Rani is eager to share her knowledge of more than three decades with all women so they can make better styling choices. In addition to the book you are reading now, *Your Body, Your Style,* Rani is the author of four upcoming books: *Your Body, Your Bridal Style: Wedding Dresses to Flatter Your Body*; *The SoulMate Checklist: Key Questions to Help You Choose Your Perfect Partner*; *Seven Types of Men To Avoid: Recognizing Relationship Red Flags*; and *Unveiling: A Celebrity Fashion Designer's Story*, a memoir of her life journey.

Born and raised in Bangkok, Thailand, Rani now happily lives in Los Angeles, California.

Learn more about Rani at www.ranistpucchi.com.

ALSO BY

ALSO BY RANI ST. PUCCHI

The Soul Mate Checklist: Key Questions to Help you Choose your Perfect Partner

Your Body, Your Bridal Style: Wedding Dresses to Flatter Your Body
(Book available February 2017)

7 Types of Men to Avoid: Relationship Red Flags
(Book available 2017)

Unveiling: A Celebrity Fashion's Designer's Story
(Book available 2017)

Learn more about Rani at www.ranistpucchi.com

Facebook: http://facebook.com/ranistpucchi

Twitter: http://twitter.com/ranistpucchi

RANI'S DESIGNS

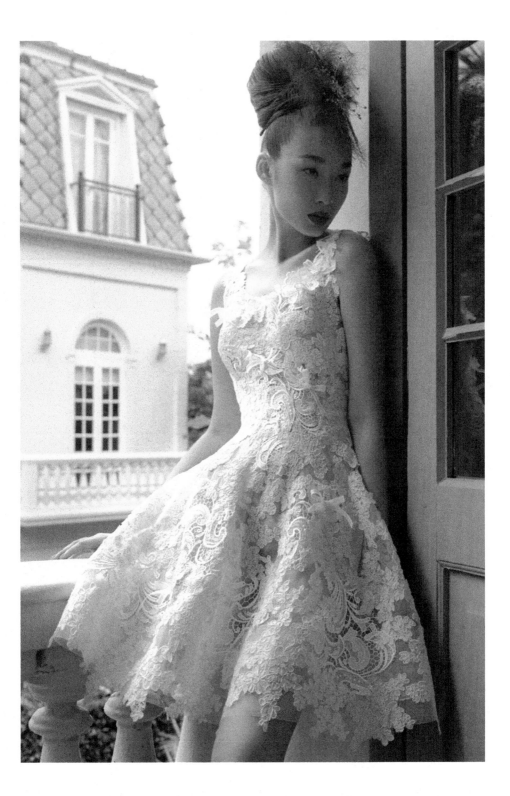

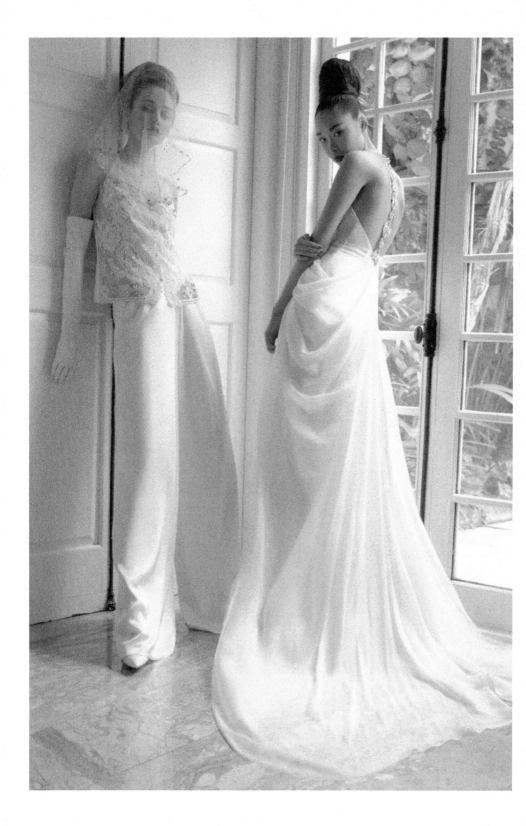

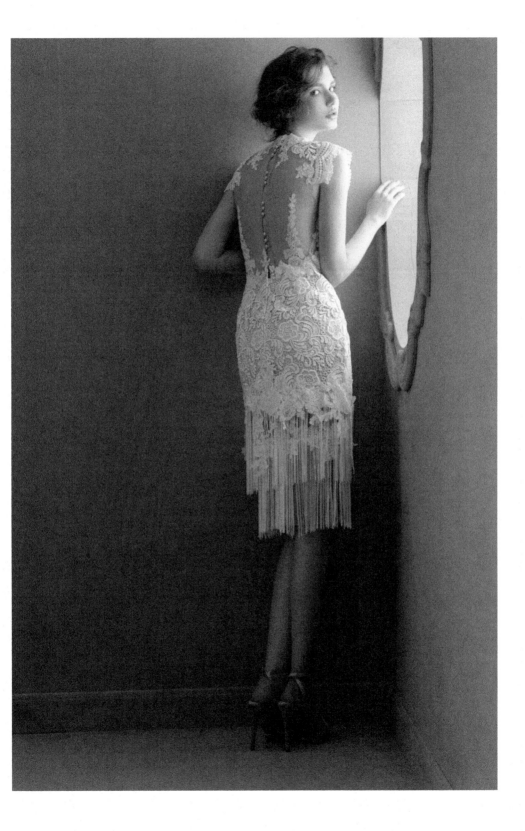

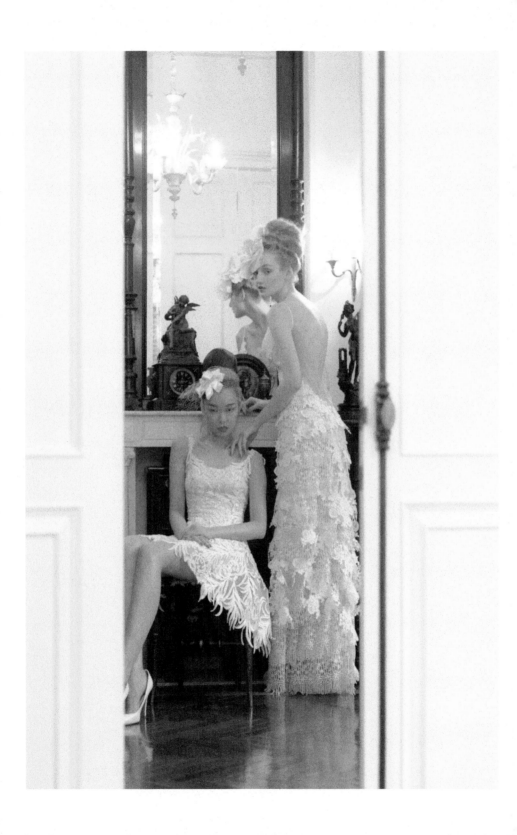

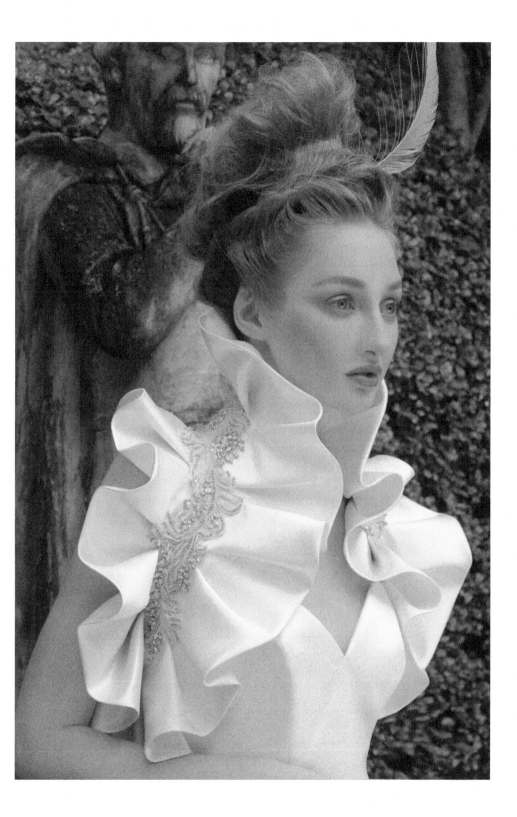

FINAL THOUGHTS

You suppose you are the trouble

But you are the cure

You suppose that you are the lock on the door

But you are the key that opens it

It's too bad that you want to be someone else

You don't see your own face, your own beauty

Yet, no face is more beautiful that yours.

~Rumi

CPSIA information can be obtained
at www.ICGtesting.com
Printed in the USA
FSOW04n0032121016
26014FS